ISBN-13: 978-1499525939

ISBN-10: 1499525931

Introduction:

What are the theories of medicine? Are there any theories of medicine that are commonly taught, understood and studied in the science of medicine? No, there are not. Medicine is about 'practice', not about theory. If anyone dares to suggest a theory of medicine, or a theory of illness, a new theory of treatment, or even an old, established theory of medicine, they will be dismissed as quacks.

All new treatment are dismissed until they meet the 'gold standard' of clinical testing. No-one mentions that the 'gold standard', of placebo controlled clinical trials, is simply a 'theory' about how to make better medicines. It is also a theory that has often been tried, and found wanting.

The field of medicine regularly uses many words that are clearly unscientific, even 'mystical'. Words like placebo, placebo effect, anecdotal evidence, alternative medicines, side effects, and remission are nonsense words that dismiss further investigation and avoid searches for scientific explanations.

There are many general theories about the cause of illness, none of which are supported by the medical community – causing more confusion.

The field of medicine has no commonly accepted theories of medicine, nor of illness, because it is by definition incomplete. Medicine is the study of holes in your health. When we use a medical paradigm to search for and study illness, we lose sight of health. When we spend all of our time looking at the holes of illness, we cannot see the landscape, nor the skies, nor the depths of healthiness.

Medicine is blind to health.

The healthicine mission is to understand health, to create and improve healthiness.

Healthicine includes studies of the wholeness of health, healthiness, and unhealthiness, as well as studies of illness and aging.

This book is a refinement and expansion concepts of healthicine as published in the book: Healthicine: the Arts and Sciences of Health and Healthiness. As I researched and wrote that book, over the course of several years, I learned to look at health, and at illness, from different perspectives.

Medicine is about the use of technologies to fight illness. Healthicine is about working with nature to create health. Health is bigger than illness, healthicine is bigger than medicine.

Tracy D. Kolenchuk

Contents

The Universal Declaration of Health

Good health is essential to happiness, and happiness is essential to good citizenship. — Charles Mayo

Health is the first of all liberties, and happiness gives us the energy which is the basis of health. — Henri-Frédéric Amiel

The Declaration of Independence states: *"We hold these truths to be self-evident, that all men are created equal, that they are endowed by their Creator with certain unalienable Rights, that among these are Life, Liberty and the pursuit of Happiness."*

Often abbreviated to: "**the right to life, liberty and the pursuit of happiness**"

Healthiness includes happiness, but happiness does not include healthiness. It is possible to be very happy, while being very unhealthy. But it is not possible to be 'very healthy', while you are very unhappy. Thus:

Everyone has a right to life, liberty, and the pursuit of healthiness.

Everyone has the right to the pursuit of 'their healthiness of choice'. There are many silly laws, and even some sensible ones, that take away these rights. We need to look at those laws in a new light, the light of health.

These rights are, as the Declaration of Independence states "unalienable rights" which are not constrained by responsibilities. It is the responsibility of the state to uphold these rights, and design laws to up hold these rights. The 'state' in its many forms, is part of our healthiness. Our healthiness does not stop at the body, nor the mind, nor the spirit. It extends to each of the communities that we create, participate in, and those that affect us directly and indirectly. Each community, from families, to schools, to churches, to corporations, to civic, state, national and international organizations and governments can be healthy, or unhealthy. Every community has a responsibility to uphold these fundamental, unalienable rights of all people.

1 Introduction to Healthicine

We begin our study of health with two close friends. Alice and Zizi have been friends since childhood. Alice is a year older than Zizi, but that makes little difference. Alice has two children. Zizi has none. They are both young and healthy. Both are happily married, their spouses are friends as well. One day, Alice and Zizi are discussing their good fortune over a glass of white wine in a local café, when Alice asks:

"How did we get so lucky, to have such good health, good relationships and wonderful families as well?"

"What do you mean by 'good heath'?" asked Zizi.

"You know," replied Alice, *"we're not sick, or hardly ever. I mean, we get a cold once in a while, but we don't have any chronic diseases, or worse."*

"Is sickness the opposite of health?" asked Zizi.

"I never really thought about it," replied Alice. *"It's an interesting question. If neither of us is sick,* **how can we tell who is healthier**? *Here we are, in the prime of our lives, strong and fit. But we don't know who is healthier. To tell the truth, I don't even know how we might begin to figure it out. What does healthy really mean?"*

"It seems we don't know much about health," Zizi replied. *"Maybe we should consult the experts?"*

"I'm beginning to see a bigger problem," Alice countered. *"There are lots of experts in sickness – doctors, there are lots of experts in fitness – Olympic coaches for example, there are lots of experts in nutrition and experts in psychology. But who are the experts in health? I can't even think of what we would call an expert in health."*

And with that, they finished the wine and agreed to meet again

3

tomorrow afternoon. Alice got the tab, and Zizi got the tip.

Alice and Zizi have discovered something important. We speak a lot about health, but know little. The words 'health care', 'health insurance', 'health clinic', seem to be about health, but are about illness. We use reductionist techniques to take illnesses apart, to trick our illnesses, to kill them, but we don't learn about, study, nor understand our health. Illness has taken over our bodies, our minds, our spirits, and our communities, so thoroughly that we call it "health". We have many medical experts, but no health experts. We measure illness while ignoring health, healthiness and unhealthiness.

It's time to study health, the science of healthicine.

What is health?

Health is wholeness. The word health comes from the word whole. Health cannot be understood by taking things apart.

Health is honest. We cannot play tricks on health.

Health is much wider, deeper, taller, and richer than illness.

The World Health Organization (WHO) defined health in 1949:

> **"a state of complete physical, mental and social well-being"**

This definition is no use to Alice and Zizi. It defines perfection. Neither Alice, nor Zizi have perfect health – they want to know who is healthier.

To study health scientifically, we need **a definition of health that facilitates measurement**. To study health in a scientific fashion, we must learn to measure healthiness. When we are healthy our health has many dimensions. When we are ill, many aspects of healthiness are present, fighting the illness, attempting to rebalance our health.

Healthicine Definitions:

To understand the concepts of healthicine, it is necessary to define some terms. The word 'health' for example is often misused by medical professionals, in Health Care (Illness Care), Health Clinic (Medical Clinic), etc. The following definitions are from a 'healthicine' perspective.

Health

Health is the measure of the completeness, integrity, and balance of all physical, mental, spiritual, and social components of a person, or a community. Illness is a part of health.

Note: We can also study the health of plants, of animals, or of the planet – but this book is about the health of humans and their communities.

Health is also a verb; To create or improve healthiness.

Healthiness

Healthiness is the status, or measurement of overall health, "a healthiness" is a specific measureable instance of health.

Overall healthiness has many components, many layers. Healthiness has many components, processes and cycles, each of which can be measured.

In theory, each component of health, and overall healthiness, can be measured – but not today, not scientifically. Medical systems are designed to measure illness.

Healthiness is about balance. Measures of healthiness are measures of balance and balancing.

Health is wholeness, all true measures of health are presented as a percentage of the whole.

Unhealthiness

Unhealthiness is the potential for improvement in healthiness. When healthiness is mapped to a percentage scale, 'unhealthiness' is the percentage inverse of healthiness.

If a health factor, or health score can be changed for the better, that potential is an unhealthiness. This concept is very important to the studies of healthiness. It also provides an alternate way to measure healthiness. We might measure unhealthiness as a percentage, and calculate the inverse to create a measure of healthiness.

This image shows the relationship between healthiness and unhealthiness. The blue line, the health score, moves up and down as your healthiness rises or falls. Your unhealthiness moves the opposite direction, by the same percentage amount.

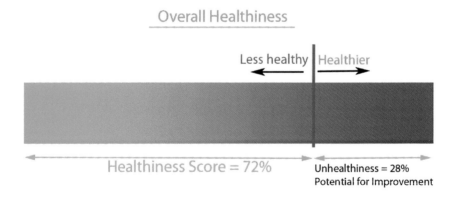

Illness

Officially, legally, illness only exists when it is diagnosed by a medical professional, although it can be diagnosed retro-actively. This is a very important concept. An unhealthiness can exist for a long period of time without being diagnosed as an illness. Unhealthiness might be measured, but cannot be diagnosed. From a healthicine perspective, illness, disease, and medical condition are identical terms – although there are some differences in different medical paradigms. They are all medical conditions that require a diagnosis to exist legally.

All illness is a part of health. Measures of illness can be used to create measures of health, but measures of illness are designed and directed towards detecting and attacking the illness. Measures of healthiness, directed towards healthiness, are poorly studied, if at all. This diagram shows an illness, or 'medical condition' mapped against healthiness.

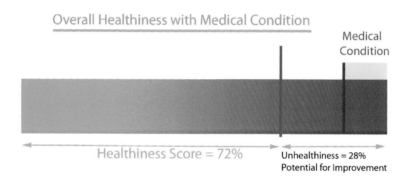

Note: The medical condition is binary, illness either exists (when it is diagnosed) or not. A bit like Schrödinger's Cat, whose state is not determined until an observation. There is no healthiness percentage associated with illness, although in theory we can develop mappings between illness and healthiness. Illness can cause positive and negative, temporary and long term changes in your healthiness.

An illness might be diagnosed correctly, over-diagnosed, under-diagnosed, or diagnosed incorrectly, but a diagnosis, the red line, is required for an illness to exist. Many employers, governments, and insurance companies enforce this requirement.

It makes sense to think that if your 'healthiness' drops too low (or your 'unhealthiness' rises too high) – you have an illness. Illness can also appear when you are, very healthy.

There are two basic types of illness, acute illnesses and chronic illnesses. An acute illness, like a cold, will pass. A chronic illness persists.

There are two basic sources of illness. External sources – over which you have little control, and internal sources over which you do have control. Most acute illnesses are caused by external sources. Most chronic illnesses are cause by internal sources, within your control.

You have an acute, external illness when you are shot by a gun, or attacked by a tiger, a parasite, a virus or bacteria. Each of these can happen independent of your healthiness rating. Each will cause a drop in your level of healthiness. Often this drop will be short term, while your body recovers and heals. When you are stricken with an external illness, a higher level of healthiness helps you recover and heal more quickly and more thoroughly.

Internal chronic illnesses are 'unhealthinesses'. Unhealthiness illnesses are a result of direct actions you might take – or not take. If you do not consume sufficient Vitamin B3, you will be stricken with pellagra. The only solution is to change your behavior.

Overall health includes *healthinesses, unhealthinesses, and illnesses.*

Remission

Remission is when an illness disappears, but the disappearance cannot be explained by the medical system. Medicine believes many illnesses as 'incurable'. Arthritis, diabetes, and many other illnesses are classified as incurable. However, those illnesses can go into 'remission', where the symptoms disappear. Remission is a mystery to medical practitioners, who don't study health. Any illness that is actually an unhealthiness, can appear to be 'in remission', when healthiness is improved. Remission is often labeled 'anecdotal evidence' which discourages investigation.

Sometimes, the unhealthiness will re-appear, as old habits re-appear, and those aspects of healthiness drop down into unhealthiness again.

Wellness

Wellness is the absence of disease or infirmity. Wellness is the opposite of illness. Either you are ill, or you are well. You might be well – but very unhealthy, or very healthy. You might be sick with an infection, or even a broken arm when you are very healthy.

Fitness

Fitness and strength are often confused with healthiness. It is possible to be very fit, very strong, and also very unhealthy. Fitness is often oriented toward specific unbalanced, unhealthy goals.

Balance

Health is not just about balance, health is about *balancing*. It's easy to confuse balance with mediocrity. The magic of health is that each individual has their own balances. Healthiness is about your ability to maintain balance in the face of challenges, and about your overall balance when no challenges arise.

Medicines

Medicines are used to fight disease. Many medicines actually decrease healthiness, tackling your health as well as your illness, under the assumption that your health will recover, but your illness will not.

Medicines that work by increasing healthiness – are **'healthicines'**. When you are suffering from the illness of dehydration, water is a healthicine, 'curing' your illness.

Some medicines tackle your illness directly, or try to trick it, like antibiotics and anti-viral drugs. One danger is that they will tackle your healthiness as well. Many drugs harm your health by design.

Medicines that only reduce symptoms allow chronic illness to progress. They can be useful as temporary measures, while planning a more effective treatment, but when used as a permanent solution, they lead to a permanent illness.

There are medicines designed to tackle 'signs' that are out of balance, on the theory that controlling certain signs can prevent illness. Blood pressure medicine aims to reduce blood pressure, with little consideration to cause or health effects.

Lastly, there are theoretical medicines. Medicines that tackle some theoretical aspect of illness, or of prevention. No-one knows the long term effects of biophospahtes, designed to 'prevent' osteoporosis, and people who take these medicines will not know the long term results for many years. Many preventative medicines, like immunizations and fluoride are in this category – not yet clearly understood.

Five different types of medicine, only the first works to improve healthiness, the only healthicines. Our medical systems do not recognize healthicines, because medicines are only measured by their effects on illness. Many medicines have been found "bad for your health" – and subsequently banned, after rigorous testing in clinical studies gained their approval. Medicines are dangerous and can distort your health, in attempts to tackle your illness.

Alternative Medicines

Alternative Medicines do not exist. All treatments are 'alternatives'.

The term 'alternative medicine' Is a marketing term. It is used by people who want to sell alternatives, and also by people who want you to 'not buy' alternatives. The FDA, when approving medicines, does not distinguish between medicines and 'alternative medicines'. Both are subject to the exact same regulations.

Side Effects

When you buy a prescription medicine, you will often see a list of 'side effects' that 'might occur' when you take the medicine.

Side effects do not exist.

Every medicine bottle has, on the label, a list of possible "side effects". This list is, frankly, a lie. There are no such things as 'side effects'. The term 'side effects' is a result of medical blinders. Medicine looks only 'ahead' as if the medicines could only drive us forward.

Medicines kill thousands of people every year. Is that a 'side effect'? Have you ever seen a medicine bottle with 'death' listed on the label as a 'side effect'?

Medicines affect your healthiness. Your illness is part of your healthiness. Rarely, if at all, do medicines only affect the illness portion of your healthiness. Medicines affect many of your healthinesses. But 'medical blindness' views the marketed effects differently from other effects and calls them 'side effects'. When a prescription medicine says "may cause X", it is an effect on your health, not a side effect. We need to study side effects, as health effects, if we are to clearly understand their effect, magnitude, and positive or negative value.

There are healthy effects, and unhealthy effects. That's it. Health effects can happen when the medicine fights illness and they can also happen when the medicine improves, or decreases healthiness.

Placebos

According to Webster's, a placebo is *"a usually pharmacologically inert preparation prescribed more for the mental relief of the patient than for its actual effect on a disorder"*. In other words, a placebo is when your doctor deliberately lies to you. Maybe your doctor doesn't know what to do, but needs to prescribe something. He knows from experience, that sometimes a placebo works best.

The words placebo, and placebo effect, illustrate one of the fundamental problems in the field of medicine – the continued use of mysticism and trickery. Placebos are when the doctor lies.

Medicine, even modern medicine, has problems shaking the mysticism. The word 'placebo' sounds scientific, but it is nothing but scientific bunk. A placebo is, as Wiki says, simply a lie from your doctor.

Either medicines work, they produce positive results, or they don't work. If we don't understand why they work, it's a learning opportunity. Sometimes, placebos work, sometimes better than medicines.

Placebo Effect

Placebo effects are real. Webster's says placebo effect is *"improvement in the condition of a patient that occurs in response to treatment but cannot be considered due to the specific treatment used"*. Placebo effects are not a lies. Medical researchers dismisses them, with an assumption that the results exist "but …not due to the specific treatment". Nonsense. The simple truth is that "placebo effects" are real effects, where we don't know what happened, or what might have caused the effects.

Many medicines have effects that are not intended by the doctor, or not understood by medicine. Researchers spend countless hours trying to avoid bumping into the 'placebo' effect. It is a ghost that cannot be exorcised. It's easy for medical science to confuse real effects with imaginary effects, making it easy to dismiss real effects. Placebo effects are thus classified as imaginary effects, ending investigations and discussions.

Placebo effects are not science. The classification of placebo effects is not scientific. Placebo effects are ignorance of cause.

In healthicine, all effects are real. Health is honest, and does not lie. It might be so complex that we do not yet understand. Your doctor might lie, and prescribe a medicine he does not believe in. But if your health changes the change is real. Only the cause is in question.

Placebos are lies. It's official. Placebos are fake medicines that your doctor pretends are real. Placebo effects are real. The only difference between a placebo effect, and a real effect is that your doctor does not believe. The question medical science needs to address is "was this effect caused by the medicine, which we thought was not effective in this case, if not, what was it caused by?" When we learn "what this effect was caused by" we will learn better ways to improve healthiness – even if the better way is to lie to some patients.

Placebo effects are most common in illnesses that your doctor cannot cure. Illnesses like arthritis, migraines, chronic pain, vague digestive problems and funnily enough – warts. If your doctor can't find the correct treatment, any treatment that works is likely to be classified with the words 'placebo effect'. "Placebo effect" simply means "your doctor does not understand what happened."

Healthicines

Actions that improve our healthiness are healthicines. Treatments that fight your illness or your symptoms are medicines. This table summarizes the differences between healthicines and medicines:

Healthicines	Medicines
Create Healthiness	Fight Illness
Improve Healthiness	Dangerous to Health
Work Slowly	Act Quickly
Not Effective in Emergencies	Powerful in Emergencies
General, non-specific	Specific to each illness
Addresses more than symptoms	Might only address signs and symptoms
Requires Personal Commitment	Requires a Medical Prescription

The right medicine might also act as a healthicine, but wrong medicines are not healthicines. Most medicines only improve symptoms of illness and are simply not healthicines. If you take them when you are healthy, they will make you less healthy.

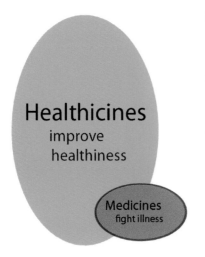

Some medicines are also healthicines, but the wrong medicine, or a strong medicine taken at the wrong time, is simply toxic.

Many medicines are bad for your health, even at the right time.

Medicine

There are many practices of medicine, from ancient systems like Chinese Medicine and Ayurveda to so called 'modern medicine', which has many fields ranging from general practice to general specialties like surgery, pediatrics, geriatrics, obstetrics, and specific specialties like , neurology, dermatology, and urology. The fields of medicine are wide, deep, and complex.

All of medicine is oriented towards illness. It is not possible to get FDA nor Medical Association for a medicine or treatment – without a reference to illness. Medicine distinguishes between wellness - an absence of disease, and illness – the presence of disease, but does not distinguish different dimensions of health. Even preventative medicine is oriented towards preventing specific illnesses – not towards improvements in healthiness.

The field of medicine uses reductionist techniques, taking apart the body, and the illness to be tackled, studying smaller and smaller portions, in the hope of winning against the illness. Health, however is whole, and cannot be taken apart, cannot be understood by taking things apart. Health can be created and improved – but attempts to reduce it to simple rules can easily lead to imbalance and illness.

Healthicine

Healthicine is the study of the arts and sciences of health and healthiness. It includes the studies and sciences of medicine. Healthicine views health, healthiness, and medicine, from a health viewpoint. Medicine views illness and medicines from an illness viewpoint.

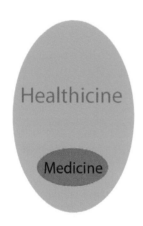

Healthicine is more than medicine. Health is more than illness. When you are sick, if you have an infection in your ear, for example, the rest of your body might see little change in healthiness.

Biology is the study of life, but biology is not goal directed. Medicine is the study of illness, with the objective of treating or curing illness.

Healthicine is the study of health, with the objective of learning about, creating, and improving healthiness.

2 The Hierarchy of Healthicine

Hierarchy of
Healthicine

communities

spirits

minds

body

systems

organs

tissues

cells

nutrients

genetics

The hierarchy of healthicine represents complexities of life and of health. Beginning with genetics, it gains complexity at each layer, from nutrients to cells, tissues, organs and systems.

The layers combine to make the physical body we inhabit. We have many cells, organs, etc. but only one body.

As we move up the hierarchy, to minds, spirits and communities we see that each of us has several minds, many spirits, and participates in many communities.

Each layer is built upon prior layers. Complexity rises at each level as more complex forms and functions emerge. Healthiness is very complex.

The concept of emergence is a key to understanding health. Aristotle said 'the whole is more than the sum of its parts'. Life, somehow, emerges from dead chemicals. Then cells emerge as those simple living chemicals become more complex. Tissues emerge from cells working together, and organs emerge from tissues. Systems emerge from cells, tissues and organs in cooperation. The cell has a body. And as life becomes more complex, another body emerges. The mind emerges from the nervous system and its integration with the organs and the body. As the mind becomes more complex, consciousness and then self-consciousness emerges, and our spirits emerge. As our cells learned to work together to create tissues, and our tissues learned to work together to create systems, our minds, bodies and spirits learn to work together to create communities. At each layer, the complexity rises. At each layer, features emerge that cannot exist in the components of lower, simpler, layers.

Healthicine is more than just body, mind, and spirit. In healthicine, we make a clear distinction between body, and mind, and between mind and spirit, based on the hierarchy concept. The body consists of the prior layers: genetics, nutrients, cells, tissues, organs and systems. Organisms with bodies – like highly developed plants – do not necessarily develop nervous systems, brains, or 'mind'. Minds is a layer above the body – and above the brains. Our minds contain the many layers of consciousness. Spirits rise above the layer of the minds. The spirits are the layers of 'will', of desire and intent. Communities emerge, taking mind, body, and spirit to a higher level.

In the fields of medicine, the concept of mind is very poorly defined. Mental illnesses are poorly classified, ranging from nutritional deficiencies or excesses (including toxicities), to illnesses of the spirit like depression and mania, to illnesses of the community like murder, war, and genocide. Spirit health is also largely ignored – due to possible conflicts with religion. Community health, and community illnesses, are barely acknowledged.

Non-Human Components

The layers of the hierarchy contain many health components that are not 'yours'. Your body contains many bacterial cells, viruses and fungi that contribute to your healthiness, but are not from your genetics. Your health depends on these components as well. If they are healthy, you are healthier. When we study at the top layer, communities, we learn that our communities include our pets, the animals we keep and eat, and even the plants we enjoy when we are walking in the forest. When these communities lose healthiness, we lose some of our healthiness.

Communities:

Communities are a natural extension of the hierarchy. Our communities can exist beyond the boundaries of the lifetime of a person or a family. Communities of science, for example, extend from before Aristotle, into the future.

Your community healthiness has two sides. You, and your communities.

Each individual has a 'community' component. Even the most self-reliant person, interacts with animals and their environment.

Each community has its own healthinesses. Communities are an extension of our life's forces. They can be healthy in many ways, and unhealthy in many ways as well. Their healthiness changes over time, just as an individual's healthiness changes over time. We need to recognize and study community healthiness and improve it.

Humans form many communities; from families to factory workers; from religious groups to politicians; from business communities to labour communities; from governments of clubs to governments of cities to governments of provinces, countries, to the United Nations and more.

Communities also permeate the hierarchy of life, and the hierarchy of healthicine. Our DNA is a community of genes, that is more powerful than any single gene. Our tissues are communities of cells, communicating and cooperating, our minds arise from communities of nervous tissues.

The evolution of our bodies, and of our brains, has stopped. Now we evolve through our minds, our spirits and our communities. It's much faster and more efficient. Someone invents an airplane or an iPhone or a Facebook, and we create communities around these new things. Our communities are the new force of evolution and a powerful force of health.

Primary Disciplines of Healthicine

The goals of healthicine are to create, improve, and optimize healthiness.

The primary disciplines of healthicine match the layers in the hierarchy of healthicine: Genetics, Nutrition, Cytology, Histology, Organ Anatomy, Systemic Anatomy, Body Anatomy, and Physiology, Studies of Minds, Studies of Spirits, and Studies of Communities.

Each layer in the hierarchy is built on the layer below. Each layer in the hierarchy is 'more than the sum of the components'. Each whole, from cells to tissues, to organs, to systems, to body, to minds, to spirits and to communities, is more than the sum of its component parts.

The primary disciplines of health are not limited to each layer or component. Each component and each layer is connected to all layers above and below. Any action undertaken to change our healthiness has effects throughout the entire hierarchy. It is important to remember that we defined these boundaries, and like all boundaries, they are fuzzy. The line between tissues and organs is not strictly clear. The line between brain and mind, or mind and spirit, is much less clearly defined.

Many of the primary disciplines of healthiness are recognized and studied by the medical profession - although from a medical, not a health perspective. Many are also studied from a biological perspective. For example Cytology is the scientific study of cells. Cytopathology is the study of cellular disease. Cell biology is the study of normal cellular anatomy, function, chemistry, etc.

What is the study of cellular healthiness? There is no word for the study of the healthiness of cells. The distinction between 'normal' and 'healthy' cells is not defined, much less studied. Does 'normal' imply perfect health? Or does it imply a commonly encountered level of unhealthiness?

The study of Systems, like the digestive system, the circulatory system, and the lymphatic system, are very weak in the field of medicine, which uses reductionist techniques to isolate system components. Cardio-vascular disease, is often referred to as 'heart disease' and the charity associated with it is the 'Heart and Stroke Foundation', not the Cardio-vascular System foundation. Health is whole, healthiness is wholeness. A focus on components, very useful when fighting illness, is not so useful in the study of healthicine. We don't want to fight healthiness.

Secondary Disciplines of Healthicine

The secondary disciplines of healthicine are created by simple combinations of two primary disciplines. We join cells and genetics to create the discipline of Cellular Genetics. Each second level discipline is an important discipline in itself. Each second level discipline has two equal sides. Tissue Nutrition is about nutrition, and about tissues. Each affects the other – and together they can affect other aspects of health. The closer we look the more rich and complex the study of healthicine becomes.

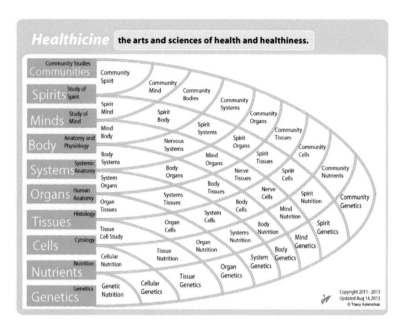

The diagram above shows the primary and the secondary disciplines of healthicine.

Many of the secondary disciplines are also recognized and studied by medical professions – due to their high correlation with specific illness. Cellular Genetics is studied in cancer research. Others, like Body Organs, the study of how the organs and the body interact to create, improve or otherwise affect healthiness are hardly studied at all as 'a complete field of study'. The medical tendency is to zero in on specific organs and study their illnesses.

Each of the second level disciplines is based on two primary disciplines – each of which can have dozens or thousands of components. The second level disciplines are hugely complex. It is very, very difficult to know what is important in each area of study. We have not studied the important questions, much less the important answers.

Genetic Healthicine

Each of the disciplines of Healthicine affects the other disciplines – everything is interconnected. Genetic Healthicine for example, is affected by nutrition, and affects our nutritional needs; our cells are based on genetics, and influence our genetics. Our genetic healthiness starts with our parents, and is extended through our communities, our choice of a mate, and through our children.

This diagram represents the field of Genetic Healthicine.

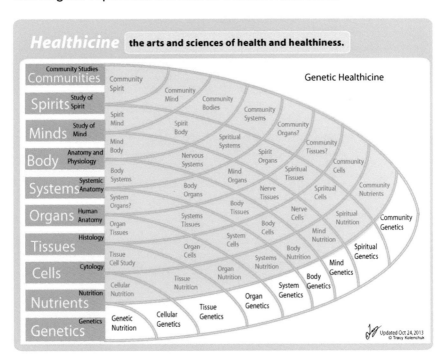

There are sub-fields of genetics that are well studied from a medical perspective, like Cellular Genetics, and some that are virtually unknown, like Spirit Genetics. To understand Genetic Healthiness we must study all sub-fields.

Nutrient Healthicine

As we move up the hierarchy, to Nutrients, we see that each sub-field can occur in two paths, as in this diagram, of Nutrient Healthicine.

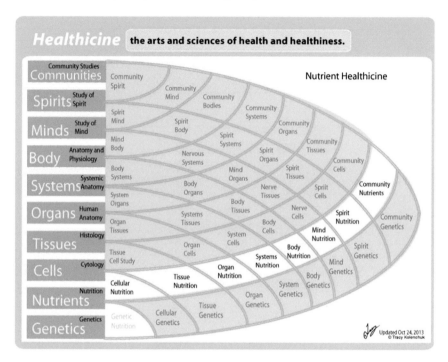

Genetic Nutrition is shaded, because it was already included in the Genetics sub-fields It is also one of the Nutrients sub-fields.

As we study nutrition, we will learn that healthy nutrients, like healthy genetics, come from diversity.

Body Healthicine

When we move up the hierarchy, to the Body, for example we see the sub-fields above and below. Each field listed in the lower-half is shaded, as it has been included in a prior category, as shown in this diagram of Body Healthicine:

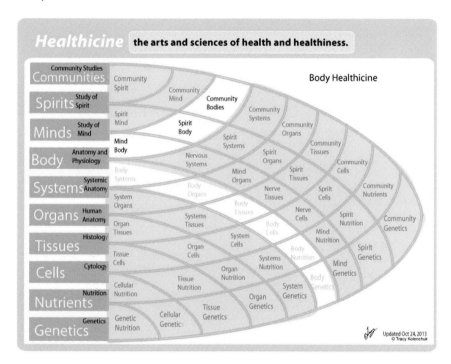

When we view the diagram for Body Healthicine, it is easy to see why we might easily assume that health is about body, mind, and spirit. Each of these components seems to be 'a person'. But the concept of body, mind, and spirit can limit our view, taking attention away from other important aspects of health, even of 'Body Healthiness'.

Spirits Healthicine

Studies of health of the mind, and health of the spirit, are currently so weak that science does not have a useful, commonly agreed upon, definition of the differences between body, mind, and spirit. This is an area that might yield the many surprises, as we explore healthicine.

Community Healthicine

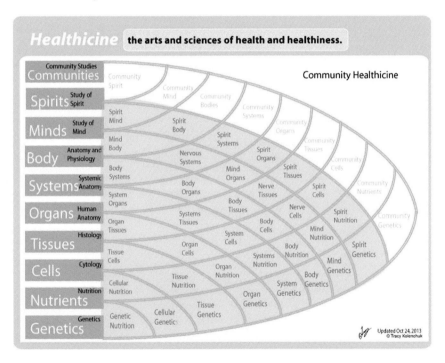

When we reach the top, we see something interesting. The sub-fields of Community Healthicine are all discovered by prior layers of the hierarchy. This might lead us to believe that we know a lot about community healthicine already. Because each prior layer extends into community – we might easily conclude there is nothing more to learn. But the opposite is true. We don't study community health, although we do study the illness of individuals in communities. Our Western focus on the 'individual' (body, mind, and spirit) blinds us to this important aspect of health.

Family is the prototypical community, our first community, with leaders, sometimes in conflict, followers – often with individual objectives, that might conflict with others and with the community. A healthy community is not without conflict, nor one consumed by conflict. Even conflict needs to be in a healthy balance.

Community begins whenever two or more beings interact. A person with a pet cat, is a community. Two people talking on the phone, or chatting on the internet, is a community. Communities can spring into existence for short time periods, and then disappear. Others, like the communities of religions, can exist and evolve and spawn new communities, for centuries.

Communities can be created, exist, evolve, grow, shrink, merge, divide, and disappear. Communities can create communities of communities.

Each discipline of community healthiness has two sides. There is the 'community healthiness' of each individual in the community, their healthiness with respect to being part of the community; and there are also the healthinesses of the community, with respect to individual members, the community as a whole, and other communities.

Our medical systems do not treat communities, thus there is no attempt to diagnose 'community illnesses'. Any illness that has a community component tends to be pushed down the hierarchy – if it is studied at all. Paranoia and loneliness are 'mental' problems. Murder, genocide, and torture, are crimes not illness.

Tracy D. Kolenchuk

3 Hierarchies of Function and Process

The hierarchy of healthicine is not just about form. Not just about the physical aspects of a healthy person. Health is more about the processes that maintain life, than it is about the elements. A dead body has all of the physical elements of the hierarchy. But there is no life, no life processes, no health – and no illness either. Minds, spirits, and communities are not so much 'things' as they are processes of life, without them, there is no life. Without life, they do not exist.

In every discipline of the Hierarchy of Healthicine, there are many functions and processes. Health is not measured by your length nor your breadth, not by your strengths, nor your weaknesses, but by how you live over time.

Health is about balance. Each of the functions of healthiness in the hierarchy must maintain balance – often within one or more cycles. When any process goes out of balance, becomes deficient, or excessive, health suffers.

Hierarchy of Function

The hierarchy of healthicine provides a framework for analysis of the processes and functions of a healthy person.

Genetics: The main processes of genetics come from the activation, repression and modulation of genes and the production of new cells. Our genetics also includes non-DNA genetic components.

Our genetic health, and healthy genetic processes, are also dependent on the genetic processes of our non-human genetics; healthy bacteria, viruses and fungi.

Cells: Our bodies contain over 200 of different human cell types and many non-human cells, each with different purposes and processes.

With over 200 different types of cells, many involved in multiple processes, we start to see how rich and complex the balances of healthiness are. Our bodies also contain many cells that are non-human, that provide valuable functions.

Tissues: Each tissue serves many functions and processes that are part of our healthiness. There are many different tissue types. Biological science groups them into four functional categories, epithelial tissues, connective tissues, nervous tissues, and muscle tissues.

Organs: Each organ serves multiple purposes. Each can be deficient or excessive. Your ear might be deficient, or excessive, or both at the same time; distracting you with irrelevant or non-existent noises, while missing important sounds.

Systems: The central nervous system is arguably the most complex system in the body, participating in all of our senses. The digestive system is very complex with to the largest number of foreign organisms involved. It is also one of the oldest systems. Hormonal systems, the respiratory system, the lymphatic system – each have unique functions that contribute to your healthiness.

Body: What functions do our bodies serve? Is it a valid question? A geneticist might say that our bodies exist to pass our genes on to the next generation, and to raise our children to ensure our genes survive. An artist might say that the function of our body is to create what our mind envisions. Others might feel, that our bodies are designed to dance; to feel free and to express that freedom physically. Our bodies and our minds require stress and exercise to keep healthy, and to encourage and enable growth and healing. We also require relaxation and sleep to allow rebuilding and re-balancing. The healthiness challenge is to know what types of movement are best for your health - and to be certain you don't overdo it. With many healthy processes - the perfect balance is not a mid-point, but healthy combinations and harmonies of exercise and relaxation.

Minds: What are the functions of our minds? Our brains sense and make sense of our environment through complex filters and feedback loops that sometimes lead to sensory illusions. Our minds remember and calculate. They can plan and predict – most obviously when we play games and predict movements and actions. The mind is conscious. The brain does not need to be conscious to function. But to be in the right frame of mind, or to be out of our minds, requires consciousness.

Spirits: What are the functions and processes of our spirits? Healthy spirits are not just balanced, they are balancing. They adjust your attitude when problems arise - and give you support. They keep you stable in unstable situations. Unbalanced spirits can result in depression, or manic states.

Individuals can consciously create new spirits and new levels of spirituality. An elephant might forget. A human can foster the 'spirit of forgiveness' in themselves and also in others through community.

Communities: Healthy communities contribute to the healthiness, and other goals of individuals in the communities, and other communities.

A healthy community supports you when you can't support yourself. And if your community self is healthy - you support your communities as well. Communities also provide ability to accomplish things that could not be accomplished by any single person. Culture emerges from communities and forms and affects communities. Culture can steer us to healthy or unhealthy directions.

Communities are the new force of evolution. Our bodies evolve very slowly, and may have reached a point, due to technological and moral issues where they are no longer subject to the push, or constraints of evolution. Our communities continue to evolve. The initial communities of family and then tribe, have evolved to the point where today's communities range from families to Facebook friends lists, to tribes or gangs and terrorist or spy cells, to local, provincial, national and international governments, to companies from partnerships, to mega-companies like Coca-Cola Company, to religious organizations and more. We create communities of communities of communities, like the Boards of Directors of the International World Bank.

In the book "**The Genius Within: Discovering the Intelligence of Every Living Thing**" Frank T. Vertosick, Jr. proposes that the evolution of life is not driven by genetics, but rather by networks – a fundamental element of communities. Networks, or communities of chemicals created life, and wrote it down in our DNA – although some life forms continue to survive without DNA. Our cells are communities of chemicals. Our tissues are communities of cells. Brains are communities of nervous tissue cells. He extends this discussion to super-organisms like communities of ants and bees. He notes that, in the same way the first forms of life wrote their text in DNA, people have evolved to write our text on paper and thus extend our intelligence far beyond single generations. However, he does not take the final step to analyze the evolution of communities of intelligent beings.

Freedom Requires Community

"Everyone has a right to life, liberty, and the pursuit of healthiness"

We need to recognize and remember that freedom does not exist without community. Individuals in conflict, or in agreement, are a community. Communities constrain freedoms. But without constraint – there is no concept of freedom. There are also no murders, no genocides, no prisons, no theft, no lies without the existence of a community. If you are the only human being on the planet, you are completely free.

Healthy communities must work to enhance rights and freedoms. We must also recognize that both freedom, and constraints can only be healthy as long as they are neither deficient, nor excessive.

Many communities have replaced healthy goals with a single unbalanced goal – to make money. This leads to many problems in our individual healthiness and in the healthiness of our communities.

Hierarchy of Processes

When life first developed, reproduction was the fundamental process. Life is about the ability to reproduce. Gradually, life developed systems for digestion, for protection (cell walls) and healing, for sensing danger – and moving away from danger. These systems evolved gradually into sophisticated coordination of cells, tissues and organs for sensing, feeling, growing and healing.

Communicating
Exercising
Reacting
Sensing
Healing
Growth

Deficient   Healthy   Excessive

Growth and healing, sensing and feeling, acting and reacting, and exercising and relaxing are all important to health. When we consider communities, we can add communicating and cooperating.

Each process can be deficient, or excessive; underactive, or over-active. These processes are active in many places in the hierarchy of healthicine. Our cells grow and reproduce and can heal, they can sense food, and danger, they can act and re-act, and work, or relax. Our bodies also grow and reproduce and can heal, sense food and danger, act and re-act, work and relax. And our communities also grow, reproduce and can heal, sense food and danger, act and re-act, and work, and relax.

Growing and Healing

When we are young, we grow tall – as we age, we might grow wider. Some parts of our bodies continue to grow, for a short time, even after we are dead. Excessive growth is dangerous, deficient growth is also unhealthy.

Healing emerges from growth and cooperation among communities of cells. When we are injured, we can grow new skin or scar tissue to protect our body. Our immune system is part of our healing system – and it too can be unhealthy; deficient or excessive.

Sensing and Feeling

Our senses emerge when communities of cells realize that food can be detected and located, and that danger can be predicted and avoided. Senses rise naturally through the hierarchy to the point where we are never certain if they are sensory, or created by our mind's predictive powers. We rely on our senses, not just to experience the external world, but also to experience our own existence. There are five basic senses: seeing, hearing, touching, smelling and tasting, but we have many other senses and sensations. We also have a sense of pain, a sense of balance. Our skin is sensitive to hot, cold, pressure, itch, smoothness and roughness. We have a sense of our body, a sense of consciousness, and a sense of self – unless we are schizophrenic, in which case we might have two or more senses of self. When we think of sensations, we find many more. We might feeling dizzy, thirsty, hungry, off balance, warm or cold, and of course, pained. We also have a "sense of place", which is derived from our communities. In one community, you might be a leader, another community – a mother, and in another, a volunteer dish washer. In each of these communities, you have a different sense of place. This sense of place affects our other senses. People in music communities hear differently and listen differently. People in dance communities, or martial arts communities, move and walk differently and have a different sense of balance.

Our senses evolve through our communities, although we are seldom aware of it. Anthropologist Maureen Matthews advises us that, "When you pay attention, it's not the individual body, it's the social body, that's paying attention, and the cultural self." Our communities, our culture determine what senses we pay attention to, and how we interpret what we sense.

Each of our senses can be deficient, or excessively active, due to unhealthiness or illness.

Our senses can also lie. We are familiar with optical illusions, but there are also sound illusions, touch illusions, pain illusions and even illusions of consciousness. Pain can be pleasurable, and pleasure can be painful.

Acting and Reacting

Acting and reacting emerge as our senses, and their ability to predict, grow in sophistication. As conscious beings we can reach beyond the simple actions and reactions of animals like our cats and dogs. We can plan our actions, and even plan to plan, evaluate our plans, revise our plans – even plan to plan to plan. We might even plan to create a planning community.

We can also plan our reactions. We can make a personal decision to not let someone, or something, cause us to lose our cool. We can consciously decide 'to get mad', or to 'not get mad'.

Exercising and Relaxing

Exercise and relaxation emerge through stretching and play to provide continuous alertness, readiness for action – and also to find time for recovery. Exercise is healthy stress. It is important to understand the meaning of stress, and the distinction between stress and distress. When we stress test materials – we subject them to opposing forces until they break. Breaking is distress. Distress must be fixed.

Stress is natural and healthy. Our health consists of many factors and many processes, constantly changing and re-balancing. Stress exists when we are out of balance, it can also move us back into balance, and can arise when we move back into balance. If we don't stress, we die.

With all processes of healthiness, health is found in balance. Deficiencies of action, exercise, lead to muscle degeneration and weakness. Excesses result in excessive stress and breakdown.

Communicating and Cooperating

Communicating and cooperating emerge naturally, as animals learn that they can provide more freedom to act, more life, more health. They emerge again as we create new communities – communities being defined by communications and cooperation. Even if one of us was the only being on the planet, there would still be communications and cooperation among our cells, tissues, organs and systems. Even very primitive single celled organisms learned to advance their species through cooperation and communications, without any sense of conscious awareness. Lichens developed when different cellular communities unconsciously learned that cooperation furthered both of their goals. As the hierarchy of life arose, each level learned the values of cooperation and communications, long before there was speech. As humans, we extend these processes to a new level, deliberately creating new communities, communicating and cooperating between them, even when we each are pursuing opposing goals.

Of course, as humans, we also developed sophisticated techniques for deceit and deliberate miscommunications. But deceit and miscommunications are not unique to humans. Even some simple plants have learned that unconscious deception can be an effective tool to advance personal healthiness.

Cyclical Processes, Functions and Balances

Healthy processes are cycles. Breathing is a simple cycle. Our sleep cycles are more complex, with many stages of wakefulness and sleepiness.

Our nutritional cycles are very, very complex. We also have many cycles based on very long timelines. Some are natural, some are artificial, some are combinations of natural and artificial cycles. We plan our work by the week, and relax on weekends. The seasons are natural cycles, and we add cyclical holidays like Christmas and Thanksgiving to each year.

The cycles of life, being born, reproducing and dying are all natural cycles of being human. These cycles are a natural part of our first community – the family.

Health is about balance, but it is balance in motion, balance within the boundaries of our cycles. Single measurements can be misleading. Height, weight, blood pressure, heart rate, temperature, all change over the time of our cycles.

Healthy Processes – Healthy Balancing

All of the activities, functions, and processes in our cells, bodies, minds, spirits, and communities, in the entire hierarchy of our healthiness can become more active, or less active - without a diagnosable illness. These changes can be healthy, or unhealthy. Our cycles naturally balance and re-balance.

As healthiness moves up and down, unhealthiness moves down and up. They are, by definition perpetually tied to each other. As we learn more about our healthy processes, how they interact, and what choices we have in their regard - we can move towards optimal healthiness, optimal freedom, and the attainment our true potential.

Creation and Art

Creation is the highest of processes. Art comes from our spirits and our communities – our culture. The healthy, sophisticated spirit creates things. Even unhealthy spirits are creative, sometimes uniquely so, because their stress pushes them further or in radical new directions.

The deliberate artistic spirit is higher than the basic spirits of consciousness. A cat is conscious and has spirit. But a cat does not deliberately create art. It is believed that the Neanderthals did not create any art. The human spirits, human processes, rise much higher than those of a cat, a dog, or a Neanderthal.

4 Signs and Symptoms

"I've been feeling a bit woozy these last few days," Alice commented.

"Are you getting enough iron in your diet? We have to look after ourselves you know…" Zizi replied.

"Oh, it's not that," Alice replied with a smile. *"It's that new guy in the office – he reminds me of Brad."*

Symptoms are observations of change. Symptoms are signs, evidence of changes caused by illness, healing or healthiness.

From a medical perspective 'signs and symptoms' are about illness.

What are signs? What are symptoms?

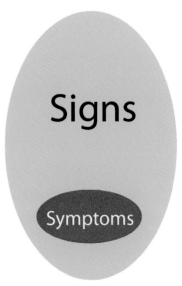

Signs are indications of healthiness or illness that can be measured objectively. Symptoms are those signs observed by the patient, some of which cannot be measured objectively. They can be measured, in the sense that the doctor can accurately state 'the patient reported symptoms of x.' Thus, all symptoms are signs, but all signs are not symptoms.

Signs are the result of observation and measurement. Your pulse, your blood pressure, your temperature are measurements of vital signs. Doctors observe and make many measurements. Lab tests measure more details, often with high precision. Signs are not about illness any more than your height is about illness. They are simply measurements.

Symptoms might be noticed by the patient or by the doctor. Symptoms are indications of change. Change can be positive and healthy, sometimes neutral, sometimes negative and unhealthy.

A symptom can be a result of:

- an actual change, or
- a change in perspective, or
- a change in observation.

One morning, we look at ourselves in the mirror and think "I never noticed that before…" We're seeing something for the first time, but we don't know if it has been there for days, weeks, even years. This can happen in the doctor's office too. The doctor might order a medical test that has never been done before – and be surprised at the result. That result might be 'part of your nature', may have always been that way, or it might be a result of a change in your healthiness.

Both signs and symptoms can indicate changes of healthiness, or illness. Signs and symptoms can be signs of growth, of shrinking, of healthiness, of healing – or of degeneration. Symptoms of healthiness are seldom discussed in medical literature, except for 'what can safely be ignored'.

It can be difficult to distinguish between symptoms of healthiness and symptoms of illness, even when we have all of the facts. If you cough, is it a healthy cough, or an illness? If you are drinking water, and it goes down the wrong way – you cough. This is a healthy cough. If you are not healthy, if you don't cough – your health can be seriously damaged. If you have a cold, and you cough, the cough is a symptom of illness. There are many more situations where a sign or symptom cannot be easily defined as a symptom of illness, or a symptom of healthiness. Even the distinction between a symptom and an illness is not clear.

Most signs and symptoms are observed with an illness orientation, and need to be re-examined to provide a useful measure of healthiness. Signs and symptoms are powerful tools in the practice of medicine. We can make them powerful tools in the practice of healthicine.

Signs of Healthiness

What are the signs of health? What are the symptoms of healthiness? There are many websites where you can enter your symptoms and get analysis of illness – but a search for signs and symptoms of healthiness fails, delivering symptoms of illness instead.

There is a simple reason for this. Illness is specific. If you have a specific illness, you will have specific symptoms. Each individual symptom of an illness might indicate several different illnesses – but when grouped together, symptoms are used to distinguish between illnesses. Health is a more general, non-specific status. It cannot be measured using the same methodology we use to measure illness.

There are many signs and symptoms of health and healthiness.

Spring fever is a symptom of healthiness. Spontaneous dance is a sign of health.

Signs of Healthiness

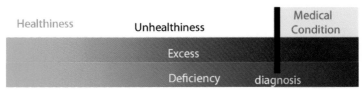

This diagram shows the gradient from healthiness on the left, to unhealthiness, to illness on the right. We all have aspects of healthiness, and of unhealthiness – and sometimes we are sick. When we are sick we might suffer aches and pains. If we are just 'of poor health', but not at a level where illness can be diagnosed, we might suffer vague, or even severe aches and pains. These might be pains of the progression of illness, or of healing. They are symptom of change.

When you have symptoms – your doctor's job is to identify the illness. If they can't find an illness they are likely to say "it's all in your mind", or "try this and see if it helps", never "it's a symptom of healthiness."

Let's suppose you are 'unhealthy', but not 'sick'. Healthiness is a scale, as in the diagram, and it is very possible to have many unhealthinesses, without having an illness. Now suppose you deliberately (or even accidently) take some action that increases your healthiness. You might notice 'symptoms' as your healthiness increases. This can happen very slowly, over the course of several months, or suddenly, over a few days. How can you tell which symptoms are symptoms of increasing healthiness, which are symptoms of healing, and which are symptoms of illness?

We're familiar with this on a small scale. If you have a cut and you put on some anti-bacterial cream, you might expect some pain from the cream, and some itching as it heals.

If your spirit is healing, you might find yourself overwhelmed by memories, sensations, and feelings. You might think you are 'mentally ill', because your symptoms are so strange. It's difficult to distinguish sensations of illness from sensations of healing, or even simple sensations of change. What might be the symptoms of a community that is healing? We tend to think of symptoms as belonging to an individual – but communities can also exhibit symptoms of illness, or symptoms of healthiness, in response to healthy, or unhealthy changes.

Healthiness is more complex than illness. We can only learn which symptoms are healthy, and which are unhealthy by taking a broader view. But this conflicts with the goals of medicine. If you have an illness, quick action is often a priority. When we have an unhealthiness – quick action might be exactly wrong, leading us to believe the problem is being resolved – when the action is only addressing symptoms, and those symptoms might be symptoms of healing.

A healing crisis can occur when you heal or detox your body, as it becomes overwhelmed by the release of toxins. The Herxheimer reaction, can occur when you take an antibiotic and your systems are temporarily overwhelmed by dead bacteria. These symptoms are not illness, they are the result of healing. But, the Herxheimer reaction can be so severe that it becomes an illness of healing.

It's difficult to differentiate between symptoms of illness and symptoms of healing. But there's a more challenging question:

What are the symptoms of healthiness? What does it feel like to be very healthy, from genetics, to diet, through every cell, tissue, organ, bodily system, body, mind, spirit and community? What are the signs of healthiness - and why don't we know?

Is it a Sign, a Symptom, or an Illness?

There is some confusion in our medical paradigm, between a symptom, and an illness, and perhaps this is to be expected. When you get a headache, it is a symptom of something. You might get a headache because your boss is stressing you, or because you are dehydrated due to over-indulgence the night before.

But if your headache continues, it becomes an illness. If it grows worse, it might become an illness with a different name "migraine", or "chronic pain". There are many cases where symptoms can be confused with illness – especially in the case of chronic symptoms, or are they chronic illnesses?

Is depression a symptom, or an illness? Maybe it's a symptom sometimes, and an illness at other times. How can a distinction be made? We should base the distinction on the cause. Once we understand the cause, it is much easier to separate an illness from a symptom.

 But finding cause is difficult, error prone, and time consuming. Many illnesses, and most chronic illnesses, have unknown causes in individual cases. Doctors often simply treat the symptoms, and do not search for the cause. When we stop searching for cause – it's easier to confuse symptoms for illness.

Is it an Illness? Or an Unhealthiness?

What are the symptoms of unhealthiness? The difference between an illness and an unhealthiness is defined by the definition of unhealthiness. An unhealthiness is a "potential for improvement in healthiness". Many so called illnesses are unhealthinesses. High blood pressure, for example. Is it a symptom, or an illness, or an unhealthiness? Usually, it's a symptom of unhealthy blood vessels, of stiff, inflexible blood vessels. Thus, the most effective, healthiest treatment for high blood pressure is to 'health' the blood vessels. Medicine often defines high blood pressure as an illness, prescribes drugs that reduce it by tricking your circulatory system into lowering blood pressure, not by healthing it. The unhealthiness is ignored, and often progresses as a result.

One of the ways to learn which illnesses are actually unhealthinesses, is to study diseases that cluster together. Those that occur together, like high blood pressure, obesity, diabetes, for example are more likely to result from unhealthiness than from external causes.

Tracy D. Kolenchuk

Measurement is the first step that leads to control and eventually to improvement. If you can't measure something, you can't understand it. If you can't understand it, you can't control it. If you can't control it, you can't improve it. - H. James Harrington

Revolutions in science have often been preceded by revolutions in measurement. - Sinan Aral

5 Measuring Healthiness

The foundation of every science begins with measurement. Without measurement, there is no science. Today, there is no science of health, because there are no measurements of healthiness.

Health is whole. A measure of healthiness is a measure of wholeness. Each measure of healthiness is mapped to a percentage scale, where 100 percent is the whole, the goal. Each measure contains the healthiness that exists, and the potential for improvement, the measure of unhealthiness.

Measures of illness are simple measurements, not typically mapped to a percentage of healthiness. Measurements of strength are also not measures of healthiness – we typically only measure strength when it is deficient, or when it is excessive. Height and weight are not measures of healthiness, unless you have a health goal.

BMI, the ratio of height to weight, is a potential measure of healthiness – although it is a crude measure. A BMI number in itself is not a measure of healthiness, because it is not expressed as a percentage of a goal. If your ideal BMI is 22.3 and your BMI is 24.5, then your BMI can be expressed as a percentage of your goal. BMI was designed as a measure of the healthiness of groups of people (not necessarily communities) and is poorly suited to measure the health of individuals, because an individual's "healthy BMI" can vary widely.

In the hierarchy of healthicine, there are thousands, no, millions of potentially useful healthiness measurements.

We must measure healthiness to facilitate optimal healthiness in individuals. Without effective measurement techniques, we don't know if any action we take has improved – or decreased healthiness; or, more likely, if it has improved one aspect of healthiness and decreased another. Today, in the field of medicine, there is no scale, there is no scientific test that your healthiness has increased or decreased - without reference to illness. We all, including our doctors, have only a vague idea of our level of healthiness.

Measuring healthiness advances the science of healthicine. If we are to learn more about healthicine - the study of healthiness, we must measure and track healthiness. We must also measure and track our measurement techniques. When we measure using different techniques, we can compare results, and improve our measurements. Until we practice measuring healthiness a lot, and make some mistakes, we don't have a good understanding of healthiness.

Measuring healthiness is hard. We notice people who are sick. People who are healthy don't stand out from the crowd. We only notice someone who is healthy if they are very old, and abnormally healthy.

Every individual has individual healthiness goals. You can change your healthiness scores by changing your health, or by changing your goals. We need to be very conscious of this complexity as we study and measure healthiness.

When we measure the healthiness of groups of people, we need appropriate goals for the group – and develop more general health goals. Individuals can use these goals to set their own goals, and 'healthicine practitioners' can use them to suggest goals for individuals. This might appear unscientific at first, but it will lead to more appropriate measures of healthiness. Health is whole – and that 'whole' has different meanings for individuals and groups.

Remember, health is not 'fast'. Illness can progress slowly or rapidly, but healthiness never changes quickly. Proposed measure of healthiness that change rapidly are probably measures of illness, not healthiness.

Healthiness Summary

Health is a general concept. A healthiness is a specific aspect of health that can be measured. Overall healthiness is a summary of all of an individual's measures of healthiness. This diagram, which we saw in Chapter 1, is a representation of a summary measurement of healthiness.

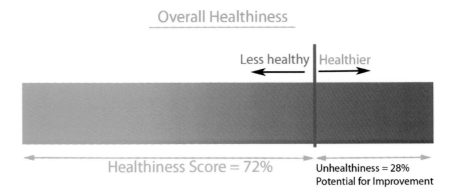

This person's level of healthiness is 72 percent. This gives 28 percent as 'potential for improvement', also named 'unhealthiness'. *Unhealthiness is not a moral judgement, it is simply the inverse of healthiness. As your healthiness grows larger, your unhealthiness shrinks. If your*

unhealthiness grows – your healthiness shrinks. A high 'unhealthy' score indicates significant potential for improvement.

Many factors of health – like hunger, sleepiness, alertness, are cyclical, having natural lows and highs over time. Some cycles are quite long – others like the cycles of breathing or pulse – are very rapid. Measurement must take the cycle into account. Sleepiness is not indication of unhealthiness if you are sleepy in the evening, but not in the morning.

There are two ways to measure healthiness. We can measure the state of healthiness, and calculate unhealthiness. Or, we can measure unhealthiness and calculate healthiness.

There are currently no standard measurements of healthiness.

There are thousands, no, millions of measurements of healthiness to be discovered. For each measure of healthiness, we need to determine what is healthy and what is unhealthy – and what might indicate an illness. There will be shades of differences, disputes and disagreements – and honest differences depending on relationships of health factors. A BMI goal might be a very different for a Quechua from Peru than a Tutsi from Rwanda.

Today, we can suggest many actions that might improve healthiness – dietary changes, physical, mental, and spiritual exercises, and community involvement – but we have no idea if the actions we suggest are appropriate for this person, at this point in time. And after the action is undertaken – we have no useful technique to tell us whether or not it was successful, partly successful, or even if it actually decreased healthiness. And if it was successful, we have no idea what next action might give a further increase in healthiness.

Can Illness be a Measure of Healthiness

Do we actually measure illness? Most measures related to illness are not actually measures of illness, they are measures of signs and symptoms of illness. It's a bit like measuring rabbit dung and footprints instead of actually catching the rabbits and measuring them.

Illness is often not 'measured'. It is diagnosed. Once it is diagnosed, treatment is prescribed. There is little incentive to 'measure' illness except in specific dimensions. The dimensions of illness that are important are:

- is it mild, moderate or severe
- is it dangerous
- how fast is it proceeding, is it growing or receding.

There is little else of importance to measure. A diagnosis is made, a treatment is prescribed. Goals are simple – to remove the illness and heal the damage. If the illness is communicable – ensure that it is contained. We don't study, nor care about the 'health' of our illnesses. We don't care about the complexity , sophistication or richness of an illness – except with regards to fighting the illness.

Health is more complex. We don't want to defeat healthiness, we want to foster healthiness. After we defeat an illness, there is still much to be done to improve healthiness. Healthiness does not 'go away', like illness. It is always there. It can always be improved.

Can we use measures of illness to measure healthiness? Yes, but not by measuring pulse rate, respiration, temperature, blood pressure or pain in a hospital setting. Health is slow. Changes in healthiness are not 'immediate' – health must be measured over time. Illness can strike fast. Health does not 'strike'. Healthiness is about balance, about steadiness.

Measures of illness, taken over time, can be converted to useful measures of healthiness. If you have a chronic illness, you can track changes in the illness over time – measuring changes in your healthiness over time. If you got five colds last year, and each lasted two weeks, we have reason to believe your health was lower than someone who had one cold last year.

Summary Health Measurements

Individual measurements of illness are not measurements of healthiness because health is about the integration and harmonies of the processes of life. Your pulse, blood pressure, temperature, measured in isolation, means little or nothing – unless you are ill. To obtain a useful measurement of healthiness, we need to measure several factors at once and view them in relation to each other. And because health is slow, we need to take measurements over time.

This diagram shows a summary of many health measurements.

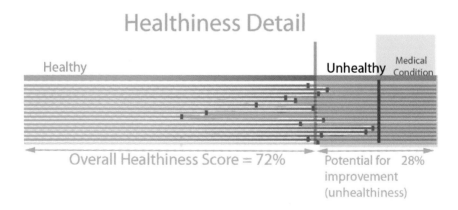

There will be lots of trial and lots of error as we attempt to make useful measurements of healthiness. We can only learn by trying.

"Measure what is measurable and make measurable what is not so."
Galileo.

How Healthy Are You?

If you and a friend, visit your doctors, and present no illness – you will receive the same answer, no actual score. Your doctor might say "whatever you are doing, keep doing it" spoken softly, or louder, depending on your age. You doctor cannot measure health, and is sometimes at a loss for words when health is encountered.

How Healthy is Your Diet

We also have no way to measure the healthiness of a food, or diet. Recommendations for improving your health are often expressed in vague, general terms: eat a healthy diet and get lots of exercise. This leads us to ask "what is a healthy diet?" and "can we measure the health of a diet?" What exercise is healthy?

If, or when, we can measure healthiness with some level of usefulness, we might be able to measure the health of a diet by the simple technique of measuring healthiness, changing our diet, and measuring our healthiness again. But we can't measure healthiness today, so that's not an option.

Can we measure the healthiness of our foods, independent of measuring our healthiness? Yes, and no. Measuring the healthiness of many foods is impossible today. We can measure the healthiness of foods, if we know what the ingredients are – but many 'natural' and many processed foods have hidden ingredients.

What would a measurement of food healthiness look like? There are two sides to the healthiness of a food. First, how healthy is the food, on its own. Can it produce healthy progeny? An egg is healthy when it can produce healthy chicks. A pig is healthy when it can produce healthy pigs. A grain is healthy when it can produce healthy grains. And second, how healthy is the food 'in our diet'. This is a separate, but perhaps more important question.

To measure the healthiness of a food, on its own, we can use the same model we use for the healthiness of people. Healthiness is a measure of how healthy it is, unhealthiness is the potential for improvement in healthiness, and illness is 'something else', that might result from unhealthiness or from external sources, as in this familiar diagram.

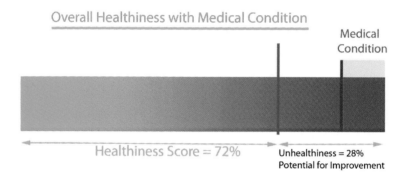

Can we also use this model to measure if a food is 'healthy in our diet'? Yes we can. The healthiness of an apple, an egg, a slice of pork, can be represented as a whole. Health is whole. That whole contains things that are good for your health – resulting in a healthiness score. Nutrients that result in health increase the healthiness score. Unhealthiness of a food would be those things that are bad for your health. If the food contains toxins, or health disruptors – those are unhealthy. Note: many nutrients become toxic in excess. If you don't need sugar in your diet, an excess of sugar can be toxic. How unhealthy is sugar? It depends on you, and on your current diet.

When we remove or lessen the unhealthinesses – we make the food healthier from a dietary perspective. What is a medical condition or an illness in a food? Illness in food is mould, rot, dangerous bacteria, etc.

Things that we would normally cut away, or remove with surgery. This results in the following diagram.

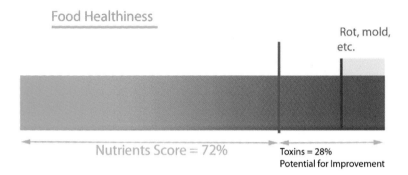

Food Healthiness

Why can't we measure healthiness of foods for our diet? First of all, in many cases – we cannot obtain the list of ingredients. There are no requirements, for example, to list all of the ingredients in many processed foods. Even foods that are not processed, like apples, can be sprayed with pesticides – but those are not on the label. Many meats are 'grown' using toxic ingredients, antibiotics, and hormones – and these ingredients exist in the meat, but not on the label.

Most of today's foods are bred, and genetically modified, grown and harvested for goals that are not related to health. It is important for 'natural foods' to survive transportation long distances to the grocery store, to look good on the shelf for as long as possible, to not over-ripen or rot quickly. These desirable qualities of food can move even natural foods away from healthiness, towards unhealthiness.

Is it healthier to eat foods that are healthier? Is it healthier to eat apples that are healthier? Is it healthier to eat chickens and cows that are healthier? We don't know which chickens or apples are healthier either, because we don't measure their health. It might be possible, although I have my doubts, that a chicken that is 'unhealthy' from the perspective of a chicken – could be a healthier food than a chicken that led a healthy life.

Are GMO foods healthier, or less healthy than natural foods? By the first measure of healthiness – can they produce healthy progeny, they are less healthy. Healthy progeny requires free and healthy results from interactions, and interbreeding, with other healthy members of the species. Technically, and legally, GMO foods are less healthy.

And by the second measure? Are GMO foods healthier in your diet? There are several factors to consider. One of the most important factors of healthiness of your diet is variety. It might be possible that a GMO food is healthier in your diet 'some of the time', but if the production of a specific GMO grain limits the variety of your consumption of that grain – it is less healthy. Secondly, many GMO foods are designed to produce specific toxins, or poisons. The more of this food you consume, the more of these toxins you consume. This is actually related to the variety issue. If you consume many different types of apples, for example, you will spread out your consumption of specific toxins that exist in apples. But when you only eat one specific variety of apple, you concentrate the toxins of that apple in your diet. Many GMO foods are taking over the market, making the entire market less healthy in general, by reducing the variety available. The third important factor in the healthiness of GMO foods in your diet is toxins. Many GMO foods are designed to tolerate high amounts of poison in their environment. These poisons are used to produce more food faster – but they are not on the label. GMO foods have higher levels of unhealthiness, thus lower levels of healthiness.

6 Aging and Infirmity

We need to learn to distinguish between unhealthiness, and aging.

Our medical systems don't measure 'healthiness', and thus don't measure 'unhealthiness'. They have no way to distinguish between unhealthiness and aging. As people get older, many get 'less healthy', but the medical system calls it 'aging'. Aging is a natural fact of life, not a disease. The word 'aging' is currently used to cover up, ignore, and dismiss many unhealthinesses.

As we develop tools to measure healthiness, we need to consider aging and infirmity. What are the differences between unhealthiness and aging? What are the differences between unhealthiness and infirmity or disability?

The difference between unhealthiness and aging is clear when we consider our definition of **unhealthiness.**

Unhealthiness is the potential for improvement in healthiness. Aging is not 'unhealthiness'. Unhealthiness can be exchanged for health. Aging cannot be changed. The effects of aging cannot be reversed. If they can be reversed – they were not effects of aging, they were 'unhealthiness'.

Effects of aging are parts of our former healthiness that we cannot change. Over time, we accumulate many slight impairments, and some severe impairments, which cannot be reversed. We call this **'aging'.**

This is an important distinction **"cannot be reversed."** If it can be changed, if it can be repaired, if it can be healed, it is an unhealthiness, a potential for improvement, a potential for better health. Mae West was wrong when she said **"You're never too old to become younger."**, you don't become younger, but you can become healthier.

If it cannot be changed – it is an impairment. If it is an impairment that was accumulated throughout your lifetime, it is 'aging'. If you are born with an impairment it is simply a disability. From a health perspective they are the same – they cannot be repaired. If you were born without a hand – a measurement of your personal healthiness should not be based on the absence of a hand. Aging impairments might be physical, like the loss of a gallbladder, or functional – like the loss of ability to hear sounds above a certain frequency.

If it can be changed, it is not aging. If we roll it back, or reverse it, it was not aging, it was unhealthiness.

If you are getting weaker as you grow older, is it aging, or unhealthiness? How can we tell? Many elderly people can regain some strength and ability through simple resistance exercises.

The part of lost health that cannot be regained is an impairment due to aging. The health that can be regained is unhealthiness. This simple concept has powerful consequences. We can only learn what is aging by trying, and failing, to change it. Once we succeed in changing a deficit, it was clearly an unhealthiness, not aging.

Unhealthiness, like illness, can also be a bit like Schrödinger's Cat , when we try to change 'aging' and succeed, we find unhealthiness, if we fail, we have found aging – until we succeed.

When charting groups of people's healthiness, unhealthiness and aging, aging is represented by black segments, as in this figure.

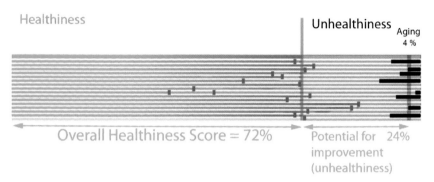

Note: because aging is 4%, the sum of healthiness and unhealthiness is less than 100 percent. As we grow older, aging intrudes on our potential for healthiness. A group of 20 year olds, has much more potential than a group of octogenarians.

Health is whole. Measures of healthiness are measures of wholeness. Each individual person is the 'whole' of themselves, and we must measure their healthiness as a whole. Thus, we don't normally include aging in a healthiness chart for individuals, because the octogenarian's score for healthiness and potential healthiness must add up to 100 percent, not 96 percent. An octogenarian has different health goals. We don't expect an octogenarian to heal as fast as a 20 year old.

When we measure the healthiness of groups, we use a different standard. If one group of people has a large population born "without a hand", that population is less healthy than a normal group.

It is important to study disabilities, impairments due to aging, etc. from a health perspective. When we measure the healthiness of groups of people, we count impairments that can no longer be reversed or changed. If a large percentage of people in a study group have impaired hearing, then this group is 'less healthy', than a group that does not have this hearing impairment.

Many studies by the World Health Organization, and other organizations, measure health by measuring impairments. This is valid for measuring the health of groups of people, but not valid when measuring the health of individuals.

When a study only measures impairments, and does not measure other aspects of healthiness – it only measures of illness. It is not measuring healthiness. If 'normal' is counted as 100 percent, we are not measuring healthiness, we are ignoring health and counting disability instead.

This takes us back to the definition of health. Health is whole. Illness is a hole in your health. Measuring holes can be done independently of measuring health. Measuring holes is not health measurement.

7 Illness

After thousands of years of medical practice, and throughout many different medical systems, there is no main theory of medicine. There are many theories of illness, but none are accepted by all schools of medicine. Why? Because medicine is about fighting illnesses, not about understanding illness.

One goal of healthicine is to develop a clear understanding of healthiness and unhealthiness, and to distinguish them from infirmity and aging.

How does illness fit into healthicine? What is illness? What causes it?

Transition from Healthiness to Unhealthiness to Illness

You don't fall ill, you slide. Sometimes very slowly, over a long period of abuse and lack of awareness. - Thérèse Bertherat

Many illnesses arise directly from unhealthiness. Normally, we don't get sick in an instant. It usually takes minutes, hours, days and even years. Medical professionals say, 10 years or more to get cancer. Years of gradual damage and over 200 changes in our cells, to grow a cancer that is visible and dangerous. What happens during this time? Your body is getting less and less healthy, for the entire time, and then suddenly, an illness is diagnosed. We think – if we could detect the illness earlier – we could fight it better. That approach only moves the point of diagnosis, it doesn't change the situation.

Some illnesses are simply unhealthinesses. They have no external cause, and can be removed by improving specific aspects of healthiness. Obesity is the most obvious example. There are many more.

Throughout our lifetimes, some aspects of healthiness rise, while others fall. When some fall too low, we can develop an illness. When we improve our healthiness, the illness might disappear. Medicine calls the unexplained disappearance of an illness "remission", does not normally investigate, and expects that the illness will re-appear. Remission is often simply "increased healthiness". And the illness sometimes re-appears when the unhealthiness, which often comes from our habits, returns. When a patient goes into remission – and believes they understand the cause, their story is typically dismissed as 'anecdotal evidence'. Medical practitioners, scientists, and researchers actively ignore transitions from healthiness to unhealthiness.

When we only treat symptoms, unhealthiness – and illness as well, can increase, as symptoms are diminished. It might appear that we no longer have the illness, but healthiness is not improved.

Illness, from a medical perspective, is black and white. Either you are diagnosed with the illness, or you are not. This concept is very important in the field of medicine. Many medicines are toxic and dangerous. It is important to have a boundary that clearly defines illness, that clearly defines when a medicine or treatment can be prescribed. Health is not black and white. To measure healthiness we need to understand the gradation from healthiness to unhealthiness. The medical paradigm, of illness and diagnosis, is insufficient for studies of healthiness and unhealthiness.

Two Ways to Correct Illness

There are two fundamental ways to correct an illness:

1. We can use healthicines that improve healthiness.
2. We can use medicines, or treatments that 'fight the illness' and allow the body to heal.

In some cases, a combination will be most effective, but often, healthicines beat medicines. Unless the patient is in perfect health (excluding the illness of course), it is unlikely that a single medicine is the best solution.

Current medical systems do not distinguish between these two types of treatment – and there is no name for this distinction. The FDA does not recognize medicines that work by making you healthy.

When the cause of an illness is slow and gradual, that the cure for that illness will also be gradual. When the cause of an illness is decreasing unhealthiness over time, the most effective treatment technique will be to improve healthiness. When the cause of an illness is rapid and dangerous, like a bacterial infection, improving healthiness is often not an effective alternative.

There is another treatment option, to treat the symptoms. This give time for further analysis – but it should never be used as a permanent solution. When the symptoms are treated – the illness is often ignored. If the illness is a result of unhealthiness – treating the symptoms allows the unhealthiness to continue and grow.

Causes of Illness

Historically, there are many theories about the causes of illness:

- **Humoral theory** states that **illness is caused by** imbalances of blood, phlegm, yellow bile and black bile.
- **Chinese medicine** states that everything, including the body, is governed by ying and yang, and **illness is caused by** improper balance of these principles.
- **Ayurveda** states that health is a state of balance between body, mind and consciousness, and **illness is caused by** imbalances.
- **Modern medicine** says **illnesses are caused by** bacteria, viruses,

genetics, toxins, and other factors.

It sounds like there is not much agreement. But there is agreement of the fundamental concepts, which we can also derive from healthicine.

Every school of medicine believes that:

"illness is caused by ..."

Or, in simpler terms, every school of medicine believes that every illness has a cause, or causes. In healthicine theory, we add the obvious, and state, "all illness is caused by too much of something, or too little of something", or, in simpler terms:

"illness is caused by imbalance, by deficiency or excess".

Health is wholeness and balance. Illness results from severe imbalance.

Arthritis, for example, has many possible causes. In an individual case of arthritis, the number of causes is much smaller. Sometimes arthritis is caused by a single imbalance, other times by multiple imbalances.

i-illness, i-disease

In Healthicine, the terms **i-illness**, and **i-disease** identify specific incidence of illness or disease. In medicine, many references to disease refer to general cases of the disease. When we search for causes of disease, it is important to distinguish between general causes of a disease – of which there might be many, especially for general diseases like cancer or arthritis – and specific instances of a disease, which have specific causes. Arthritis is a general term for many diseases, that have many possible causes. But if you have arthritis, your i-disease, your i-arthritis, has specific causes. If we are to find the best treatment for your i-disease, we need to find your i-causes.

Simple Illness

A simple illness is an illness that has a single cause. We often search for the cause of an illness as if all i-illnesses have one cause, and we often expect illnesses to be treated with one cure, as if they have one cause.

Simple illnesses are rare.

They are rare because they are the easiest to recognize, diagnose, treat and prevent. Many illnesses that we think of as simple Illnesses are actually complex.

Complex Illness

A complex illness has more than one cause. There are many more possible complex illnesses than simple illnesses. Most illnesses are complex. All chronic illnesses are complex.

There are 13 vitamins. A severe deficiency or excess in any one can result in a simple illness. How about a 'not so severe' combination of deficiencies and excesses in two or more? There are over 12 billion possible combinations of vitamins that might lead to illness at a level that would not cause an illness from a single nutrient imbalance. That's just from vitamins – there are over 100 nutrients known to be essential to healthiness.

Our bodies are remarkably good at maintaining balance, at creating and maintaining health. But our medical sciences are remarkably impoverished in their ability to measure imbalances and use those measurements to determine the causes of a complex i-illness. Science is flush with studies that show statistical correlation between individual nutrients and illness – but the analysis seldom goes further. Someday we might be able to create a health profile for any person, and study how each individual's profiles relate to their specific healthiness, unhealthiness, and i-illness.

You might be suffering from many unhealthiness, from several different imbalances, from mild to severe. Which are most important? Which are contributing to your illness? Much of today's 'health advice' uses the shotgun technique. If you try to do all of the things that are healthier, you can avoid illness – in theory. This is not only very inefficient, it is impossible. There are many 'tricks' to avoid arthritis, heart disease, etc. Health is honest. You cannot trick health.

Six Classes of Illness

We can group most illnesses into six classes of cause: genetics, nutrients, toxins, parasites, growth and stress.

Genetics - we are each conceived with a specific genetic code. In some cases, this genetic code is faulty, leading to illness, sometimes very quickly, and sometimes after a very long time. Genetic factors can be deficient - where the person does not have genes to avoid an illness, or healthy, or excessive - where the genetic factors have a negative effect on the person's health. Diet and exercise can affect the activation, deactivation and impact of many genetic factors. Diet can also provide us with, or deny us access to the genetics of healthy bacteria.

Nutrients are a key to health, and also a key to illness. Many essential nutrients have corresponding deficiency illnesses. A healthy intake of nutrients leads to healthy cells and a healthy body. Even essential nutrients can cause illness in excess. The most challenging, and important question about nutrients is 'what is optimal' at this point in your life'. Illness caused by specific nutrient deficiencies or excess are easily diagnosed if they occur in the short term. Long term, or combinations of nutrient deficiencies or excesses are more difficult to understand, diagnose, and treat.

Diet is a key to healthiness and to illness.

We have some control over our diet, but we're never certain what is in our foods. Some ingredients are within our control, but many are not.

Toxins often cause illness. In addition, all nutrients are toxic in excess. Many toxins are contained in foods – even in natural foods. Toxins can also be absorbed through the skin and from the air as we breathe. When we have an infection, or other health problems, our own bodies or the bacteria, can generate toxins. Industry creates new chemicals daily - it is very difficult to learn which might be fast, or slow toxins. Most toxins come through the foods we consume.

Parasites, bacteria, viruses, etc. - are one of the most commonly cited causes of illness. You can suffer from a parasite deficiency or a parasite excess. Your body is host to healthy bacteria, fungi, and viruses. Some can cause illness. Some can be healthy in some people, in certain circumstances, and unhealthy in other people, in other situations. Many common parasitic illnesses, like norovirus and salmonella, are spread through food.

The healthy bacteria in our digestive systems are complex ecosystems that can vary widely in composition over time, and from person to person.

Cleanliness works to eliminate parasites. But, the definition of a parasite is not perfectly clear. Because many parasites contribute to our healthiness, killing them decreases our health. A bacteria that is healthy for one person might be very unhealthy for another, even someone closely related. Health is not simple.

Growth, includes our immune systems and our healing systems. Our bodies are well adapted to dealing with health imbalances. We have systems that protect us and heal us. Sometimes these complex systems make mistakes. Our bodies require healthy immune systems and healing systems to deal with the stress of day to day living. If these systems are deficient, as they often are elderly people, unhealthiness can creep in – leading to illness. Alternatively, healing and growth can also become excessive leading to other illnesses. Obesity is an unhealthiness of growth.

Stress is the final potential cause of illness. Too little stress, specifically in the forms of physical and mental exercise - can turn our muscles and brains to mush. Healthy stress is and vital to health. Some people use the word 'eustress' to refer to good stress, and 'distress' to refer to bad stress. Excessive stress can lead to physical or mental illness and even to broken bones. Some people can be motivated by levels of stress, that might be painful for others, or at other times in their lives.

Technically, we could view most unhealthiness, most imbalances, as 'stress'. Nutrient deficiency, toxin excess, etc. are all stressful.

Illnesses, in each class of illness, might be an unhealthiness, over which we have control, or an external illness. We can control some genetic factors through diet, and others in our communities, through our choice of a mate. Is stress and internal cause, or an external cause? Of course, both are possible. Stress happens. Sometimes many stresses happen at once. On the other hand, we have quite a lot of control over our stressors, if we choose to exercise that control.

Dietary Illness

When we look at the different classes of illness, it is clear that our diet, the foods we eat and the foods we don't eat, have a huge effect on our health, and also on our illnesses. Diet is a key, to illnesses in every class.

But have you noticed... When you go to visit a doctor – in most cases – you will not be asked about your diet. Why is that?

Chronic illnesses are even more likely to be caused by diet than short term illnesses like colds and influenza. But if you have a chronic illness, how many doctors will offer a dietary analysis?

Our medical systems consistently fail this aspect of healthiness and it's not hard to deduce why. Our medical systems want to sell us medicines, not food. If a food is the solution to your illness – your doctor and the medical companies can't make money curing it. It's even more challenging if the solution to your illness is to stop eating something. Can they sell "don't eat that"? It's not for sale.

Dietary analysis is difficult and time consuming. Have you got time for healthiness? There are many reasons why dietary analysis is difficult, – and including the fact that patients lie about their diet, consciously or unconsciously. As well, in many cases, we have no idea about the ingredients of our foods.

Community Illness

What about community illnesses? Are community illnesses, like violence, vandalism, murder, war, and genocide a different class of illness? A tendency towards risk taking, including vandalism and violence, is a contributor to the health of our genetics, by forcing us to leave home as we enter adolescence. Many health factors, many causes of illness are healthy sometimes – and unhealthy in other situations or from other viewpoints.

Chronic Disease

A chronic disease exists when we are unable to identify or treat the cause. If we can successfully treat the cause – the illness is no longer chronic. There are several reasons why we might not be able to treat the cause:

- We cannot find the cause. Most chronic diseases have thousands of possible causes. It can be very difficult, and very time consuming to identify all of the relevant causes in a specific i-disease.
- The patient prefers the cause, and the disease, to the treatment. A long term smoker, suffering from coronary artery disease, might continue to smoke even after suffering a stroke. The cause can be more important to the patient than the illness, which has 'already struck'.
- The cause is gone. If a finger joint is crushed in a door, the cause is gone – but damage might never completely heal.

One of the reasons our medical systems cannot find the cause of a chronic illness is due to the difference between healthicine and medicine. Medicine does not measure, or treat healthiness nor unhealthiness. Many chronic illnesses are actually chronic unhealthinesses, thus are not able to be cured by medical treatments designed for illness. Medicines are not effective treatments of unhealthiness, because they do not increase healthiness. In many cases medicines reduce healthiness, and can make chronic illness worse over the long term.

Because it can be so difficult to identify the cause of a chronic i-disease, most doctors, and most medical textbooks recommend treating symptoms. It is much easier to succeed by treating symptoms. Treating symptoms can be very profitable. Finding and treating causes can be very expensive, and frustrating for the doctor and the patient.

We need to learn to health our chronic diseases. We need to find better techniques to root out i-disease causes, and better ways to heal the damage done by old injuries.

Chronic diseases can only be successfully treated with healthicines, not by medicines. Even the medical textbooks agree, by grudgingly describing many chronic diseases as 'not curable' (by medicine).

The best Treatment for Illness

The most effective tool to fight illness is health.

The first tool we should use to fight illness is health. Health can be improved before illness is diagnosed. Health can be improved after illness is diagnosed.

Tracy D. Kolenchuk

8 Diagnosis

Diagnosis is horribly complex. For every illness, every diagnosis, there is a diagnosis failure rate. Illness can be diagnosed correctly, incorrectly, over-diagnosed or under-diagnosed. Sometimes you might go to a doctor, but no diagnosis is received. In some cases, even a correct diagnosis does not help find the best treatment.

Diagnosis gives us a 'name' for the illness, but in many cases, the name does not provide any indication of cause, and thus provides no direction towards the most appropriate treatment.

Because many i-illnesses are the result of unhealthiness, and medicine does not study healthiness, causal diagnosis is problematic. Medicine names the disease, and use that name to identify the treatment. The healthier path is to find the cause. The same disease can have many causes, but each i-disease has a smaller set of specific causes. When we view diagnosis from a healthicine perspective, we see that we must identify specific, not general, causes of illness, to improve healthiness.

Many diagnoses ignore causes of illness. It is too much work, too difficult to identify the cause. It is time consuming – and in medicine, time is at a premium. Health however, is slow. We have time to search for health – we will still be here tomorrow unless we have a mortal illness.

Diagnosis by Medicine

Suppose you have strange set of symptoms. You visit the doctor. The doctor doesn't know what it is. This cluster of symptoms could indicate several different illnesses – and there might not be a test that can make a firm diagnosis. Or the test might have significant risk. What is a doctor to do?

Prescribe a medicine. If it works – it was right (or it doesn't matter). If it doesn't work, try something else. At least one of the alternatives has been eliminated. Diagnosis by medicine is a very effective problem solving technique. If the treatment worked, and that was not the correct diagnosis – who cares? Does it matter? The illness is gone.

There is another common scenario. The doctor might simply prescribe something to treat the symptoms. Our bodies are very effective at healing themselves. In many cases, a prescription that addresses the symptoms makes the illness less troublesome – and the body heals.

This is diagnosis by medicine. We can do better.

Diagnosis by Healthicine

For many illnesses, the most effective treatment is an increase in healthiness. Medicines act quickly, and healthicines act slowly. This tells us which illnesses are best candidates for diagnosis by healthicine. Diagnosis by healthicine is most effective for:

- i-illnesses where the cause has not been identified
- i-illnesses which act slowly, over long periods of time
- i-illnesses where the recommended treatment does not actually cure the illness.

There are many illnesses that fit this description; arthritis, heart disease, Alzheimer's, many cancers, and many others.

Can the doctor prescribe an increase in healthiness? No. Today, medical doctors cannot actually prescribe an increase in healthiness. It's against the rules. Prescriptions must be based on a diagnosis – and there are no recognized diagnoses for unhealthiness. All medicines must be 'effective against illness' to be approved by the FDA. There is currently no approval process for a medicine or treatment that improves healthiness. As it should be – we can't use medicines to increase healthiness, we use healthicines.

To prescribe an increase in healthiness we must be able to measure healthiness, not just illness. We need to learn which of the many unhealthinesses, that are present, are contributing most strongly to the illness and the risk of illness.

We are a long way from a systematic ability to diagnose by healthicine, far away from an ability to prescribe healthicines instead of medicines.

Treatment by healthiness has an interesting bonus. If an increase in healthiness is prescribed, and the problem goes away – we have the same result as 'diagnosis by medicine'. We don't know what happened. We're not sure if the diagnosis was right, we're not sure if the medicine helped.

The difference? The patient is healthier. Not just 'less sick', healthier.

Tracy D. Kolenchuk

9 Preventing Illness

Health is key to prevention. If it makes you healthier, it prevents disease – if it makes you less healthy, it contributes to disease.

Don't be confused by 'statistical preventatives'.

The first key to prevention of illness is healthiness. If you want to prevent illness, improve your health. Increase your strength, balance, integrity, security, creativity and your communities. Which area needs the most attention in your life? In your health?

The second key to prevention is health maintenance. If you are healthy – you need to "keep doing what you've been doing." It's all too easy to slide backwards or spiral down. Health does not look after itself.

For many illnesses, healthicines are the most effective medicines, they are also the most effective preventatives.

When you are ill, fight the illness. When you get sick, it's time to see a doctor. Wellness is important.

Healthiness is more important. Healthier people get sick less often and recover faster. But they will get sick. Sickness is part of healthiness.

When you are not sick, you can't fight the "non-illness", and many attempts to avoid illness are superstitious nonsense. The best way to avoid illness is to improve healthiness.

The Preventative Test

Does red wine prevent heart disease? Doe aspirins prevent strokes? Does fluoride prevent tooth decay?

If you study each of these questions, you will find that the research is inconclusive. The problem is in the question. When we take random actions to prevent illness (or create random justifications for our wine consumption), we risk putting our health out of balance, and the results will be random as well.

For prevention, we need to ask the right question. It's not worthwhile to research the wrong question – even if a 'statistically significant' result is found.

The right question: **Does it improve healthiness?**

Does red wine improve healthiness? It's a difficult question, that has not been asked, much less studied, much less answered. It is likely that some aspects of red wine can make us healthier, and other aspects can decrease our healthiness. Thus, the answer to "does red wine improve healthiness" depends on the individual, as well as their current states of healthiness and unhealthiness. Our current model of prevention assumes that 'things' are either healthy, or unhealthy. This is simplistic, and dangerous.

The danger, in our current model of prevention, is that we will become less and less healthy, as we work harder and harder to avoid illness. Has this already begun to happen? How can we tell?

10 How to Create and Improve Healthiness

How can we improve healthiness? First, know that health is not 'illness'. We often use 'tricks' to fight illness. We cannot 'trick' health. Of course we can sometimes trick ourselves into healthier actions, but that is not tricking our health.

To create healthiness, to improve healthiness, address fundamentals of health: balance, security and integrity, strength, creativity and community.

Health is about balance, and ability to re-balance in the face of adversity. When we are young, we are vulnerable. We need security and community to support us. As we grow older we need integrity in ourselves and our communities to reach and maintain our health potential.

We need to create. Maslow called this 'self-actualization'. We sing, we dance; we create songs, we create dances. We paint, we write. Creativity is an indication of healthiness. Unhealthy people destroy things, sometimes themselves and their communities.

The malleability and empathic powers of our brains enable sophisticated mental processes. We are born without language, without morals, without the ability to survive. We learn from our communities, and create new communities.

Our healthiness extends from our genetics and nutrients to our cells, organs and body, through our minds, spirits and communities. Healthiness encompasses all that we are as individuals and all of our communities.

Healthocratic Goal

The Hippocratic Oath was developed by the field of medicine, over 2500 years ago. One of its most quoted phrases has been translated as:

"I will prescribe regimens for the good of my patients according to my ability and my judgment and never do harm to anyone."

Doctors need to promise to "do no harm", because many medicines, many treatments "do harm". It could be argued, that the entire purpose of the field of medicine, is to "do harm to illness". Many of the goals of medicine are to eliminate illness entirely – but we have learned, through the indiscriminate use of antibiotics for example, that dedication to goals of destruction is not healthy. Destruction is about creating imbalances, and making things fall, making things fail. Health is about creation and beauty and balance.

It is up to the doctor to determine if a treatment does harm, or does more harm than good on a case by case basis. Today's doctors are often restrained, or forced, into specific treatments once a diagnosis is made. Our medical system does not allow the doctor to decide, except by changing the diagnosis, and can actually force doctors to "do harm" if certain diagnoses are made. Medical associations, insurance companies, marketing forces, do not consider individual patients needs. As a result, they find it easy to 'do harm' and to justify harm. They don't take the Hippocratic oath.

We might update this oath using knowledge of healthicine. An update of the medical oath has been attempted before, and the World Medical Association (WMA) adopted and recommended an updated version in 1948. There is another important oath, the "Oath and Prayer of Miamonides". An update is not what is required. We need a different goal. These oaths are valuable historical medical documents. But they are missing what is most important in healthicine. They are oaths by doctors, to be used when treating patients. But healthicine is not just about sickness and death. When we lift our head up from the work of a doctor, to view health and healthiness – we see a more valuable goal.

"to create and improve healthiness"

When we study the creation and improvement of healthiness, and make that our goal, we see that many aspects of the 'medical oaths' are only important when we are so sick that we need a doctor. The healthicine goal is relevant when you are healthy, and it can be more relevant when you are sick.

This healthocratic goal applies not just to doctors and their patients, but also to healthy people and their teachers. It is a goal of individuals and communities, from families to faiths, from companies to corporations, from lawyers to lawmakers and from governed to governments.

Health is often not improved when we fight illness, it's up to your body, your health, to heal you after the illness is defeated. Health is created and improved when we set out to create health. The best preventative of illness is not a prophylactic, not a medicine 'just in case', it is the creation and improvement of healthiness.

The first step to creating and improving healthiness is simple, make our goal, the goal of healthicine, to:

"create and improve healthiness"

Creation is a much more powerful act than destruction. It requires all of our knowledge, integration of our intelligences, communication, cooperation – and a quest for beauty. Destruction of illness is a difficult challenge, but compared to the creation of healthiness, it is simplistic and trivial. Medicine measures itself by the death of patients. We must learn to measure the health of our people, our communities, and our environment.

Can we Improve Healthiness?

Health is about wholeness, and wholeness is about balance. To improve healthiness we use balance. This chart shows some ways to improve healthiness in some of the layers in the hierarchy of healthicine. We can quickly see that each layer's healthiness can be improved by consumption, and also by abstinence.

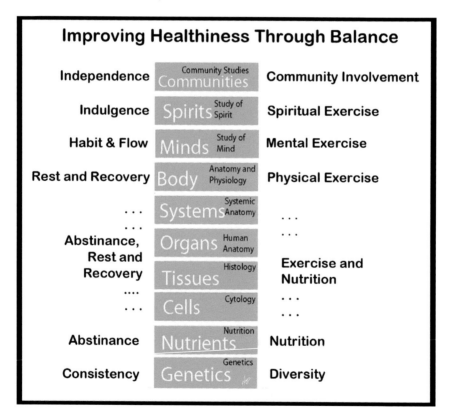

This shows what we already know . There are many ways to improve healthiness. Improvement is a change – if we wish to improve our healthiness, something needs to change. It is important to know both sides of change. When we think of medicine, we think of something we 'take'. Health is about balance, not just consumption. Sometimes we need restraint more than consumption.

The main entry points to improving healthiness are: Nutrients (abstinence and nutrition), Systems (rest and exercise), Body (rest and exercise), Minds (habit & flow and mental exercise), Spirits (indulgence and spiritual exercise) and Communities (independence and community involvement). Nutrition is important – so is abstinence. Exercise is important – so is rest. This duality pervades the hierarchy, because health is about balance. Each time we move from imbalance towards balance, our healthiness rises higher.

Improvement is change.

You can "change your mind", for example. That phrase has two meanings, both important. You can make a decision and change that decision: changing your mind. On the other hand, you can make a conscious decision to 'change your mind', to change the way you perceive and react to the world. The small book: "**The Compassionate Brain: How Empathy Creates Intelligence**" by Gerald Huther Ph.D. discusses how our minds develop and how we can deliberately make plans and take actions to 'change' our mind, not just your thoughts. This is a very powerful concept, perhaps even a step above the simple concept of 'freedom of choice'. Sometimes the best thing way to health your mind, is to simply let it flow, rather than making it work.

There are many things we can do that change our spirits. Of course techniques to improve spirits health includes diet and exercise. The wrong foods can make you depressed, and lack of exercise can drain your will to live and to act. Our spirits arise from our 'wants'. Healthy, balanced spirits, balance indulgences and restraint.

Community involvement is important. It's also important to be independent, to exercise our independence. Communities can even improve the independence of individual members. Both communities,

Tracy D. Kolenchuk

and independence can be healthy, or unhealthy, depending on the individual circumstances. When we change our communities, we can change our health and the health of our communities. Our communities also affect our healthiness. Communities create belief – and if we believe we can become healthier, it happens. With belief, the alcoholic can become sober, and with community, stay sober. Communities that are unhealthy can become healthier, but first, the members must learn, and understand that some things are unhealthy, especially when excessive or deficient. Then, they must believe that the community can change, not just the individuals. Communities are very rich and complex. We might change our relationships with our family, our immediate community. We might get a pet. We might choose to participate actively in a commercial or political community – or to terminate an involvement that is depressing our health. We are social animals. The concept that community activities can improve our health is so ingrained that it is almost invisible. We speak of friends and pets lifting our spirits, as if it was something we just learned. But, we have kept dogs as pets for over ten thousand years.

There are four important factors to consider if you want to change your health for the better, and one important concept: freedom.

First, we are all individuals. Everyone is different, has different diets, different types and levels of exercise, different social or community environments and involvement. There is no 'one size fits all' to improve healthiness. The most effective way to improve an individual person's health depends on the individual and their current health status.

Each community is also an 'individual' community. Some communities are made up of many individual communities, each of which are made up of many individuals. The most appropriate way for a community to improve its healthiness is unique, although there are useful general concepts; honesty, openness, fairness, communications and cooperation, etc. that make communities healthier.

Second, once you undertake an activity to improve your healthiness – your healthiness changes. Once it changes, the most effective way to improve your healthiness is a different technique.

Third – health is slow. Health cannot be tricked by 'easy solutions'. Tricks are 'tricky'; more likely to exchange one illness or unhealthiness for another. We need honesty to create health. Health is not 'how we feel today', it is 'how we are'. If we are sick, but we have a healthy diet, and a healthy body, healthy minds and spirits, and healthy communities – the illness will not last. The inverse is also true. If we are well, not sick, but we have an unhealthy diet, unhealthy body, unhealthy minds, spirits or communities – our wellness will not last.

Fourth, and finally, consumption is often not the best way. Consumption alone creates imbalance, creates unhealthiness. Marketers fill the shelves and our heads with things we can buy to improve our health. But every entry into the hierarchy of healthiness has two sides. If we are deficient in nutrients, it's important to eat. In many cases, it's important to abstain. We need to exercise and we need rest. We can stimulate our brains with activity or caffeine, and we need to sleep. We are social animals, we need to be involved in our communities – and we need down time, quiet time, time to be alone and contemplate our navels, or look out the window.

Consumption and abstinence must be balanced and harmonized.

There is one other important concept to be taken from this diagram: freedom. If we are to improve our healthiness, we need to have many choices available. In many cases, the key to finding balance is something new, something we are 'missing', even if the thing we are missing is abstinence. The key to finding balance in health, is to expand our choices. Actions that limit choices, limit freedoms and limit our healthiness.

Communities often limit some freedoms, and create additional freedoms through community actions. But beware of communities that actively work to limit the freedoms of individuals or other communities.

Diet and Exercise for Health

When your diet is wrong, medicine is of no use. When your diet is correct, medicine is of no need. -Ayurvedic Proverb

Diet and exercise are the most effective ways to improve our health. We've known for many centuries. But what diet? What exercise? Most of today's recommendations for diet and exercise are designed to fight illness, not to improve healthiness. Some are designed to create imbalances in strength – for example, athletes in competitions.

We often think of a diet as 'cutting back' and exercise as 'doing more', but often the opposite is needed. It's very easy to fall into a deficient diet, where it is necessary to supplement or eat more of different foods. And it's also possible to drift into exercises that hurt your health – perhaps most common is lack of sleep. Watching television at night can be an unhealthy exercise.

The Science of Nutritional Healthiness

There is no science of nutritional health. Today's science of nutrition is a science of sickness. You can search for nutritional health, you will find platitudes. Eat healthy food. Which foods are healthy? Eat real food. Eat a variety of food. Check out the 'food plate'. X is bad. Y is good. For every nutritional recommendation, you can find a condemnation.

What's going on? The science of nutrition, is totally directed against illness. Red wine is 'healthy' because it prevents cancer (statistically). Fat is bad because it makes you fat (they say) and therefore ill. Search and research, but you will not find any information about foods that make you healthy, only about foods that make you more, or less likely 'statistically', to get sick. You might find food that claims to make you healthier, but proof is lacking. We cannot, do not, measure healthiness – so there is no way to make a scientific statement about nutritional healthiness. The USFDA enforces this rule by requiring ALL health claims to make reference to scientific studies of illness.

We measure tendencies towards illness with infinite precision, but we don't measure healthiness. A science of human nutritional healthicine does not exist.

The Science of Supplement Healthiness

As you try to study health, you might encounter the 'supplement' debate. The supplement debate is not about science, it is about illness and dollars. Mostly dollars. Those who sell medicines, don't want you to buy supplements. Those who sell supplements, want you to buy.

Supplements, like foods, are studied from an illness perspective. Do they prevent illness X? Do they cause illness Y?

We cannot measure healthiness, thus, we cannot measure the healthiness, nor the unhealthiness of supplements. Neither side of the supplement debate has science in their corner – it's up to you to make your own decisions, and maybe that's for the best. What you need is freedom to decide for yourself.

Tracy D. Kolenchuk

11 The Failing Edge of Modern Medicine

Is your doctor healthier than you? Clearly, medicine has a blind spot.

Health.

The Science of Medicine

The science of medicine spends all of its time searching for illness, treating illness, preventing illness, helping people recover from illness. This constant focus on illness is a powerful tool to help those who are ill, and those who might become ill. However, the focus on illness makes the field of medicine blind to health. This blind spot, like the blind spot in our eye, is invisible. It moves as our vision moves from illness to illness. Hiding in plain sight.

According to Wiki (Wiki's definitions can change at any time), the field of medicine is a field of "applied science", a discipline of science that applies existing scientific knowledge to develop practical applications. This is not science – it is simply use of scientific results to produce technologies and products, with 'sales potential'.

The fields of medicine are widely varied, controversial and often adversarial. Conventional doctors distrust chiropractors, grudgingly accept osteopaths but maybe not naturopaths. Faith healers are dismissed as 'placebo effect'. Shamanic practices are often illegal, whether their technologies work or not is irrelevant. We ridicule witch doctors – while attempting to emulate them by creating new drug secrets combining obscure, often poisonous ingredients, and controlling the dose to control the danger. Ayurvedic medicine is similar to fields of medicine that have been discarded by conventional doctors – yet it persists because, frankly, it works. Sometimes, it works when conventional medicine fails. Traditional Chinese Medicine practitioners confuse them all, using a complex system, and a long history of success. Acupuncture, one of the practices of Chinese medicine is not understood despite repeated studies by conventional medicine – where many claim it is impossible, or 'placebo effect', conveniently forgetting that placebo effects are real effects.

The Failing Medical Paradigm

"Did you hear about Tom?", Zizi asked.

"No, what happened?, Alice queried.

"He had to get rescued. He went up into the mountains with those climbing friends of his. They're not mountain climbers – they call it 'scrambling'. No real equipment except for warm clothes and a good set of boots.", Zizi continued, *"Anyway, they were scrambling up a mountain – as they have done many times before. Tom is the strongest climber, so of course he wanted to go a bit further when the group stopped for a rest. He kept climbing."*

"Did he fall?", asked a worried Alice.

"No, that's not how it went. He was doing real well, but, you know – it can be harder to get down than to climb up. He couldn't see a way down, so he kept climbing. Before long, he was trapped. He moved higher and higher – but he couldn't find a way down. Eventually, a rescue team had to be called, with ropes and climbing equipment, to bring him down the slope."

"Interesting. I've never heard of that before," Alice commented.

"Me neither," Zizi confirmed, *"but, apparently it happens on a regular basis. There are many places where it's easier to keep going up than to come back down."*

Modern medicine has progressed steadily over the centuries, but in the past few decades, progress has slowed – in some cases, it has stopped, in some, it even appears to have reversed.

Have we climbed up a ridge, in the wrong direction – such that we are now unable to return to home ground, to common sense?

The United States of America spends more money per capita on illness than any other nation, but is consistently ranked well below the top 20 nations in medical care. There is lots of activity, but the evidence, and the overwhelming trend is clear. Many aspects of modern medicine have grown past the boundaries of efficiency and effectiveness. Beyond the boundaries of healthiness. Modern medicine has grown fat, rich, and lazy. It has grown unhealthy and ill. Has it been trapped by its successes?

The evidence is to be found in the concept of i-disease. An i-disease, or an i-illness, is a specific case of a disease. Many disease names are general, covering a wide class of causes. But if we are to find effective preventions, and effective treatments, we must identify the specific i-disease and treat it. When medicine treats symptoms instead of causes, it is treating a general class of illness, not your specific disease.

When we find a cancer, for example, no-one searches for the cure. Proof? When an i-cancer is found, no-one searches for a cause. There is no attempt to determine if addressing the cause will address the i-cancer. Even those who might claim to 'cure cancer' do not search for the cause in individual cancer cases. When i-cancer is found, the next step is often "cancer panic". Even cancers that are very slow moving, like prostate cancer, are often treated with "cancer panic", with a medical paradigm, not a health paradigm. We have decades to study the effects of health on prostate cancer, but no-one is studying healthiness.

There is blame. There are lots of researchers, in theory, searching for causes of cancer. Meta-studies abound, and the results suggest that everything causes cancer. And everything seems to prevent cancer as well. The medical paradigm in action. When we study healthicine, we will learn the cause of most cancers: unhealthiness.

If you have a cancer, you have a specific disease, not a general disease. You have one i-disease, and the cause can be found in your body, in your life. But if you have cancer, no one will search for the cause. If your i-cancer is serious, treatment is important. But if the i-cancer is not causing immediate danger – it may be more effective to search for the cause. Once cancer is diagnosed, medical science gives up searching for the cause. How can we expect to find the cause if we don't study individual diseases?

There are many illnesses where modern medicine has given up.

Arthritis is classed as a disease that is incurable. Even the community groups, like the Arthritis Foundation make statements like "You are the key factor in **living successfully with** OA (Osteoarthritis)" and "Today, an estimated 27 million Americans live with OA, but, despite the frequency of the disease, its cause is still not completely known and there is no cure." They do close with "The Arthritis Foundation leads the way in helping people with arthritis live better today and create better tomorrows through new treatments, better access and, ultimately, cures."

If you have arthritis you have a specific incidence of i-arthritis with specific causes. Arthritis has many, many causes, but your i-arthritis does not have many causes. If you are suffering from a slowly progressing i-arthritis, you can donate money to 'find a cure', but no-one will help you to search for your individual causes – to find your i-cure.

The American Diabetes Association makes similar statements. They even give advice on "Living With Diabetes". Suggesting that you "Enroll in the Living With Type 2 Diabetes program and let us guide you through your first year with type 2 diabetes." There is not a hint of a cure, and not a hint of a cause – much less a suggestion that you might search for your i-causes.

Diabetes progresses slowly. There's lots of time to find the cause in individual cases. But the medical paradigm is searching for a cure. The cure is healthiness. And to find healthiness requires finding the cause, not some random percentage cause – the specific causes of specific cases. Your i-diabetes has only your i-causes. If you find them, you can slow the progress. Sometimes, you can stop it, even reverse it.

With the exception of fundraising efforts, modern medicine has given up on cancer, diabetes, and arthritis. Medicine has given up searching for 'causes of individual cases' of many illnesses. There are only misdirected searches for 'cures'. There is more time spent 'searching for a cure' than is spent searching for each patient's causes.

You cannot find a true cure for any 'chronic illness' if you cannot identify the specific causes in individual cases. But, it's not cost effective to search for individual causes. Many chronic illnesses can also cause permanent damage, damage for which there is no treatment, no cure.

Arthritis, and diabetes are only two of a large number of illnesses where medicine has not only failed, it has given up. There are many more. Make a list of 'chronic diseases' to begin a list of many medical failures.

These illnesses result from progressive unhealthiness. Medicine does not study healthiness, cannot measure individual unhealthiness.

There is no money to be made (today) in improving healthiness, so there are no attempts to improve healthiness.

Treatment vs Cure

Many dishes many diseases, Many medicines few cures. —
Benjamin Franklin

Because we have so many diseases that are 'incurable', like arthritis, diabetes, and chronic pain, we have 'progressed', in many cases, from 'cures' to 'subscriptions'.

What are the top selling drugs, or medicines? The list of top selling drugs for the past decade reveals a simple fact. Almost NONE of the top selling drugs cures the disease being treated. Instead there are 'subscriber drugs'. You sign up for life and learn to live with the disease, the drugs, and the side effects. There is lots of money to be made in 'not curing' an illness.

Both conventional drugs and alternative products use the same approach. Drugs used on chronic disease do not cure the disease. They are designed, tested, and marketed to deal with symptoms of the disease, not to cure. There are alternative practitioners who succeed in curing some chronic i-diseases, by improving the health of the patient. But they are largely ignored, and their techniques, and even their results, are often shunned by the medical establishment.

Insurance companies have adopted the same model. If you have a disease like cancer, or arthritis, or diabetes, your medical insurance will pay for treatment. But it will not pay for a cure. Insurance companies recognize the 'facts' put forward by the medical establishment (they are part of the medical establishment) and the illness support foundations – that there are no cures. If you do find someone cures your disease – it does happen – your insurance company will not pay for the cure – unless it's on their list.

We know how to cure

We know how to cure arthritis. We know how to cure cardiovascular diseases. But we're not doing it. We know how to cure cancers. Conventional doctors are not allowed to cure many diseases. There are people who have cured their cancer. They dismissed as 'anecdotal evidence'. Their cases, their real results, are ignored, not studied, not even acknowledged by the medical professions, as their ranks grow.

The search for a "cure for cancer" is outside the boundary of modern medicine and the limits of today's medical methodologies. But the fundraising continues, because fundraising can be successful, even if the search proves impossible.

There are many diseases that cannot be 'cured', they must be 'healthed'. The cure for cardiovascular disease is not more drugs, not more statins, it is to health the circulatory system. When we think about it, it only makes sense.

But we don't know how to 'health' an illness. We've never tried. There are no scientific studies.

The Medical View

Why is this happening? How are illnesses diagnosed? How are medicines designed and tested? Not by illness nor by cause. By symptoms.

Symptoms are the key. Our medical system searches for signs and symptoms of illness. If the patient does not have the defined signs and symptoms – then illness cannot be diagnosed. This powerful technique can lead to powerful errors in healthiness.

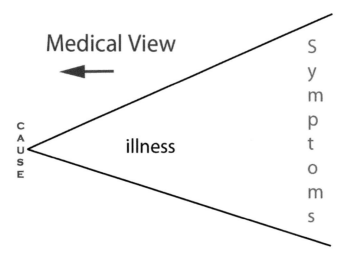

Symptoms help to identify the illness and guide the search for the cause. If the cause is removed, in many cases the body recovers from the illness, and the symptoms disappear.

But for many illnesses, our medical system does not look for the cause. The focus begins and ends with symptoms. We call these 'chronic illnesses'. They are simply the illnesses that we have not yet learned to analyze, to understand, to treat, and to cure.

We have sophisticated diagnostic and measurement techniques for signs and symptoms. We detect 'illnesses' earlier, and this has become one of the mantras, or goals of modern medicine. When you visit your doctor, you might be told you are well – or that you have an illness. Your doctor might even warn you of an oncoming medical condition or illness. The medical view is very powerful.

When we can find the individual cause, we usually have the ability to cure. But if we can't find the cause, the normal course is to treat those symptoms that are most disruptive. Sometimes we rename the illness, or create an illness, named after the symptoms. For example, a pain that continues for more than 6 months, becomes classified as a 'chronic pain', which is no longer a symptom, it is a disease. Rename the symptom as a disease, and treat the symptoms, not the actual illness, not the actual cause. Success is easier when treating symptoms – and the patient can 'feel' the results.

When we take a drug for our symptoms, the illness still exists, and in many cases is still progressing, but the symptoms are fewer or less noticeable. This is a chronic illness.

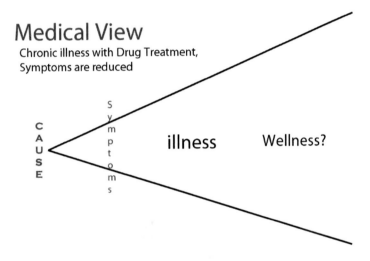

Medical View
Chronic illness with Drug Treatment,
Symptoms are reduced

illness   Wellness?

In this diagram we see the symptoms reduced, as a result of a drug treatment. The cause still exists – exactly the same. The illness and the cause have not changed. They might even grow more severe over time. Only the symptoms have been reduced. Our medical systems focus on symptoms judges the illness as 'reduced', because the symptoms were reduced. But the illness has not changed at all. Is this 'wellness'?

The Healthicine View

The healthicine view looks for healthiness over symptoms. Suppose you have a headache.

You can take a painkiller, a medicine. The medicine will reduce your health to the point that you cannot feel the pain. The medicine does nothing to make you healthier. If what you need is time to recover, it is an effective technique. Remember that medicines act more powerfully depending on the dose, and also acts quickly.

If the headache was caused by last night's alcohol overconsumption, you are dehydrated and your dried out brain is shrinking and crashing into your skull ever so slightly. Drinking water is a healthicine. It improves your healthiness, and your headache goes away. Notice that the healthicine takes time and it is not 'powered by dose' – drinking too much water can actually give you a different headache. Healthicines are about balance.

If your stress is causing your headache, controlling your stress, or controlling your reaction will reduce or eliminate your headache. There are many healthicines for a headache, but many, like drinking water – are dependent on the cause. Medicines often appear to work regardless of the cause, because they do not address the cause, they work against symptoms.

Natural solutions for your headache might be healthicines, or medicines, and sometimes it's difficult to tell, because some natural solutions might not be understood. Cayenne and almonds are minor painkillers - medicines. Yoga and regular exercise are healthicines. Is feverfew a healthicine or a medicine? Maybe it depends on the cause. Avoiding coffee is a healthicine if your headache is caused by excessive caffeine.

Of course, if your headache is caused by a brain tumor, none of the above solutions is valid, you need to see a doctor.

The healthicine view looks in the opposite direction of the medical view. The medical view zooms in, like a microscope, or telescope, to find the specific illnesses hiding in the body. This technique is very effective for some illnesses. But for the healthicine view – we need to turn our viewpoint around. Instead of looking for small, hidden illnesses or symptoms – we need to view health as if we are standing on the edge of a huge valley – with all of the majesty of nature spread out before us. The majesty of health.

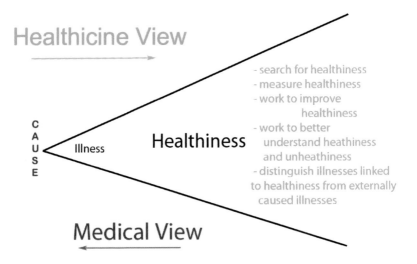

The healthicine view looks for healthiness, not for illness. It recognizes that a chronic illness is actually a lack of healthiness, the presence of unhealthiness. The way to treat unhealthiness is to improve healthiness.

When some people cure their cancer, cure their arthritis, cure their diabetes they don't fight the illness, they don't fight the symptoms, they improve their healthiness – and the disease disappears.

The healthicine view agrees with the medical view when the cause can be identified. But when the individual cause is not identified, healthicine has three priorities:

1. Improve the patient's healthiness.
2. Continue the search for the cause.
3. Treat the symptoms if necessary.

Treating the symptoms first – the common medical approach blocks the search for a cause, by making the symptoms and the illness less visible.

Treating symptoms first, promoting drugs that only treat symptoms, gives up on the illness, gives up on the cause, and gives up on the patient. Treating symptoms first encourages ignorance of the actual causes of the i-illness.

Unhealthiness vs. Illness

Modern medicine fails, when it encounters unhealthiness, and continues to search for illness.

When a 'medical condition' is actually a 'health condition', modern medicine, both conventional and alternative medicine, still use the "medical model".

Sometimes, illness comes from a single cause, as in the previous diagrams. However, in many cases, illness is a result of extended, complex, or severe unhealthiness. Many, perhaps most, i-diseases have aspects of unhealthiness, and aspects of illness. We might like to think of obesity as a 'health' condition, and of cancer as an "illness" condition. We might be wrong on both counts. We might think that sloth causes obesity. It is more challenging to think that obesity causes sloth – and maybe more important. As we study i-disease in detail, we might learn that these views are correct in some cases, but incorrect for other i-diseases. Until we learn to study health, we cannot know.

Medicine, modern medicine, does not study healthiness, does not pursue healthiness, does not even acknowledge healthiness nor unhealthiness. As I write this, healthiness is not in the dictionary. Our medical systems view health as a binary state – either you are healthy, or you are sick. Health is perfection. On-line dictionaries that contain the word 'healthiness' simply refer, or link, to 'health'.

Good applied science in medicine, as in physics, requires a high degree of certainty about the basic facts at hand, and especially about their meaning, and we have not yet reached this point for most of medicine. — Lewis Thomas

Moving from Illness to Healthiness

Many medical systems, work to move individuals from illness to wellness. As soon as you are well, as in 'not ill', attention turns away. It's time to expand our vision, expand our horizons, expand our goals and objectives. We need to move from illness to wellness, and from wellness to healthiness. If we aim for healthiness, we can go directly from illness to healthiness.

We need to expand our view, our goals, our actions, in the fields of medicine, and healthicine. We need to move beyond medicine, beyond treatments, beyond products, beyond the doctor, and beyond those systems that constrain us today. Of course when we do that, it's no longer just medicine. Healthicine is much more than medicine.

It's time to move beyond illness beyond wellness, towards healthiness. Healthiness includes illness, it includes wellness, and more. Illness will always be with us, but when our sights are set on health, much of today's illness will become a remnant of the past.

It's time to move beyond the studies of medicine, towards the studies of healthicine. To move our focus from illness to healthiness.

It's time to move beyond medicines, to healthicines. Medicines only treat illness. Healthicines create healthiness, losing many illnesses in the process.

It's time to move beyond the study of signs and symptoms of illness – we need to study the signs and symptoms of healthiness, of which signs of illness are one small part.

Our medical paradigms are very powerful and very effective at treating some illnesses. But there are many illnesses where they perform poorly and many cases where they cause more damage than health.

It's time to study health, to study healthicine. There's a lot to learn.

12 The Arts and Sciences of Healthicine

We should not expect the arts and sciences of healthicine to be 'finished'. If we are to learn about health, we need to study health. There's a lot of work to be done; a lot of mess to be made, and some beauty to be found.

The Science of Healthicine

Today, there are no PhDs of health, no philosophers of health nor healthicine. No scientists studying healthicine.

There are thousands of medical research journals, but not a single journal of health. There are many scientific journals with the word 'health' in their titles – but medicine as their goal.

There are many fields of study in medicine. None of healthicine. It's time for a change.

Today, there is little wisdom with regards to health. The field of medicine often uses the word health, but studies illness exclusively. Current study and knowledge of health is driven by illness and by commerce; a quest for insights that make money – not a quest for understanding, wisdom or health.

Healthy Illnesses, Unhealthy Medicines

Tis healthy to be sick sometimes.   - Henry David Thoreau

Medicine judges all illness as bad, and absence of illness as good, a simplistic and incorrect assumption that leads to misunderstandings when we try to create and improve healthiness.

Our medical paradigm does not acknowledge the concept of 'healthy illness'. We have already noted that some symptoms are symptoms of healthiness. It's time to acknowledge the next layer: some illnesses can be indications of improving healthiness. Some illnesses can result in improved healthiness.

In an overgrown, dry, dying forest, a forest fire gets rid of dead, unhealthy undergrowth, facilitating new healthy growth. Forest fires are fast and symptomatic. They are symptoms and results of a crisis of severe unhealthiness that is a natural result of unrestrained growth. They flare up, like an illness, and then fade after the dead wood is gone. Healthy growth follows slowly, after the fire. The forest is sick for a while, then healthier afterwards.

There is at least one illness that many have compared to a forest fire, maybe many more. Influenza is a curious illness. A virus attacks cells and causes them to die. Normally, influenza burns itself out. It's as if a normal influenza virus can't attack healthy cells, only ones that are old or weak. And after you have the flu, new cells can grow to replace the unhealthy cells.

This theory is not well studied. Our medical systems treat influenza as a deadly disease, even though virtually no-one dies from it. We cannot measure, or know, if flu makes any, some, or most patients healthier afterwards, until we can measure health.

If influenza is a healthy illness, then what's the flu vaccine? An unhealthy medicine? We don't generally take time to ask if medicines are 'healthy' or not, although we know that most medicines are toxic.

Until we take healthicine seriously, we will not understand which illnesses might be healthy, nor which might be unhealthy, which medicines are healthy, which might be unhealthy.

Scientific Studies of Healthicine

Someday, we might see a published, scientific research paper that measures change in some aspect of healthiness cause by a specific action on a test population. A clinical study of a specific health technique or product, that measures a healthiness of a group of subjects , none of whom have been diagnosed with any illness, then gives some of them a placebo for three months, and others a health product. And at the end of three months, measures again – and finds a significant difference in the health (there was no illness to measure) of the subjects who were not on the placebo.

Is this possible? Not today. We have no scientifically accepted measures of any specific healthiness, much less for overall healthiness. And there appears to be little interest or activity towards the development of useful measures of healthiness. There is no science of healthicine today.

Today's clinical studies limit their view to studies of illness. Many limit their view to studies of symptoms of illness. One or more symptoms are measured. Then a treatment is applied – and the symptoms are monitored. Observations that are outside of the symptoms being monitored are classed as 'side effects'. Nonsense. All 'side effects' are actually health effects. But we don't study health. A scientific study of healthiness would monitor and document all effects, all observations – positive, negative, even those that are not understood, that we might learn to understand them in future studies.

In archeology, scientists are not able to understand every aspect of every finding. They have found a solution. Only a small part of each finding is examined in detail. The rest is documented, and preserved for future analysis, under the assumption that future analysis will not only have more time – it will bring more knowledge to the table. We need to use this technique in the study of health. Medicine often ignores facts, classifying them as 'anecdotal evidence' and throws them away.

Sometimes worse, it views facts as proprietary, owned by private corporations, not by the community humans. How can we expect to learn about health if we throw out the evidence? How can we progress when research results are hidden more often than published?

Are you healthy?

Are you healthy? It's a challenging question. Healthiness is a complex scale, not a YES/NO. When your doctor does your checkup and proclaims you healthy, what does it mean? Doctors search for illness, not for healthiness. If no illness is detected, you are 'well', but that says nothing about your healthiness.

Doctors cannot give you a score for your 'wellness'. Wellness is the opposite of illness – but it is not the 'presence of wellness' any more than an absence of elephants signifies the presence of 'non-elephants'.

Have you known someone who had a good, or even excellent medical checkup, but was struck by a severe illness shortly afterwards. That unhealthiness was probably present at the time of the checkup.

Our ability to measure tissue unhealthiness, that might lead to cancer, for example, is very poor – perhaps non-existent. Our medical establishment does not even entertain the concept that tissue unhealthiness, that can be measured, leads to cancer. If they did, tissue healthiness would be measured, and we would be able to take steps to improve tissue healthiness – and to measure the improvements. But we're not even sure what 'tissue healthiness' actually means. So weak our knowledge of health.

We work so hard to 'avoid illness', that we also avoid healthiness.

Your doctor might tell you that you are healthy. You might believe you are healthy. But how healthy are you? No-one knows. No-one knows how to measure healthiness, and today, no-one is trying to learn.

The Science of Health Measurement

The most challenging, the most important question in the field of healthicine is "how to measure healthiness". If we cannot measure, there is no science. We might discuss, argue, agree and agree to disagree about how to measure health – that would be progress.

The field of medicine is huge, infinite. Healthicine is more infinite.

Once we begin to study healthicine – the challenge will be to learn which actions will bring us the most healthiness. This requires many measurements of healthiness.

Healthicine is so new, that we will have difficulty finding the right questions – before we can look for the right answers.

It's time to smell the coffee, and wake up to health. As we do, we will realize that healthiness is not just a science, it is also an art – we need to bring all of our creativity into play to learn about, to understand health, healthiness, and healthicine.

In the field of medicine, creativity, and play, can be dangerous. Medicines are dangerous. Medical techniques are often avoided until danger is imminent. Medicines are fast and tricky.

Health is slow. Health cannot be tricked. Health, and healthicine requires creativity, even play and playfulness, if we want to progress.

Tracy D. Kolenchuk

Conclusion:

"I wonder," Zizi asked, *"who are the experts in health?"*

"There aren't any," Alice replied.

"Surely some people are experts in health. What about Dr. Oz?"

"He's an expert in illness. No-one studies health – independent of illness. No-one can tell which of us is healthier, when we're not sick."

"What about fitness experts?" asked Zizi. *"Don't they make us healthier?"*

"They might work to make people healthier, but they have no scientific tools to measure overall healthiness. Like weight loss experts, they are willing to sacrifice health for specific goals they believe are healthy."

"But aren't strength and agility measures of healthiness?"

"Measures of health are measures of balance, not of excess. Strength and agility might be in balance, in harmony with the rest of your body – or deficient, or in excess." Alice countered.

"What about nutritionists? Surely they study health?" Zizi asked again.

"Nutritionists are not scientists. Give a nutritionist three potatoes, that do not have any disease, and ask 'which is healthier?' Don't hold your breath waiting for an answer. Your nutritionist has no science on which to base any measurement of healthiness. Is the organic potato healthier? We see this debate often. Why is it a debate – because there is no science. No-one measures the health of your food, without reference to illness. There are many theories of healthy nutrition – but there is no science. There are no health experts."

"Hmm… ", Zizi thought out loud, *"maybe we should become the experts? Where would we start?"*

"I'm not sure we can, it might require a whole new way of thinking."

Thinking about healthiness requires practice. Our medical paradigms are firmly established, and they constrain our thinking. To understand healthiness, we need a healthicine paradigm. We must to force ourselves to ask questions about health, not just about illness.

Today, health improvement, or decline, is not relevant. Health is not measured by doctors, and doctors cannot issue prescriptions for healthicines.

In our initial studies of healthicine, it may be important to stay as far as possible away from illness and disease. Although illness, disease and medicine are a part of healthicine, turning our attention to illness is a distraction in the search for health. It deceives us into thinking we understand, just because we can produce 'medical' results.

The exceptions are diseases that are misidentified by our medical system. Diseases that arise directly from unhealthiness, like high blood pressure, diabetes, arthritis, and many cancers. These types of diseases need to be studied from our new perspective. Our current perspective is failing us when it encounters these types of illness.

When you want to think about healthicine, you need to ask different questions. Simple questions like: "How does this relate to health?" Let's make an example of a very common discussion about illness, and look at it from a health perspective.

The common cold – a medical perspective:

- How can we prevent the cold?
- How can we prevent spreading cold germs?
- How can we treat the symptoms?
- How soon can we recover?
- Is there a cure for the common cold?

The common cold – a healthicine perspective:

- Does the common cold attack people who are healthy, or people who are unhealthy?
- What aspects of healthiness, what measures, when deficient or excessive, make us more susceptible to the common cold?
- Which symptoms of a cold are symptoms of illness?
- Which symptoms of a cold are symptoms of healthiness and healing?
- Is it healthy to treat the symptoms?
- After you recover from the common cold, are you healthier, or less healthy, than before the cold?
- Does the common cold make individuals, and communities, healthier, or less healthy?
- Is it healthy to never have a cold?
- What is the healthiest thing to do when you have a cold?

The questions that arise from a health perspective might seem foreign, even silly to someone who is stuck in a medical paradigm. We need a health paradigm to help us understand health.

A Healthicine Paradigm

In the medical paradigm, health is, like the spirit, unknowable, untouchable, immeasurable. We look to illness and disease first, distorting our vision with the ugliness of disease.

A healthicine paradigm looks to health first. A healthicine paradigm searches for beauty.

What might we find when we adopt a healthicine paradigm? What might we learn?

In the beginning, a healthicine paradigm will extend our current knowledge. In the end, it will turn some of our current knowledge on its head. Some of our medical knowledge is on its head today, and needs to be upended.

In the end, we will learn to create healthiness, to create and enjoy the sensations, and the beauty of health.

Acknowledgements:

I would like to thank the following people, who provided advice, assistance and encouragement in this project.

Andy Whiteley and Ryan Mullins - Wakeup-World.com

Sayer Ji - Founder: GreenMedInfo.com

Dylan Charles – WakingTimes.com

Allan Beveridge

Jonathan Drachenberg

J. Michael Drabiuk

Marshall Melnychuk

CPSIA information can be obtained
at www.ICGtesting.com
Printed in the USA
LVIC06n0128260915
455845LV00002B/7

* 9 7 8 1 4 9 9 5 2 5 9 3 9 *